EXPLORING AROMATHERAPY

PROPERTIES, ENERGIES & AROMAS

Barbara Christensen, CA

How to use the properties of essential oils in your daily routines.
Or as a part of your business or energy practice.

Exploring Aromatherapy / Barbara Christensen. -- 1st ed.
ISBN: 9781792170577
Imprint: Independently published

What you believe, is already yours.
What you desire, you already have.

This is what having my family has taught me beyond anything else.
We have everything inside of us, and around us to live our best life.
We are our only obstacle, and we are our greatest asset.

There is no way that I could actively seek the knowledge of alternative
wellness without the support of my loving family. I dedicate this book
and this smile on my face right now, to them.

Awareness is the first step in healing.

— DEAN ORNISH

CONTENTS

1

EXPLORING AROMATHERAPY

I am honored that you have decided to discover the amazement that essential oils can have on your mind, body and soul! Now is the time for you to enter a zone, or dimension if you prefer, that makes you happy and healthy. My goal, as a Certified Aromatherapist, is to help you understand the properties and possibilities of essential oils, and how they can change the way you live your life. These oils have this sort of magic power to make things smell better, taste better, and after diffusing I often find that colors look brighter and sounds seems more appealing. That is what makes essential oils such a fantastic area to expand your knowledge.

The first time I was introduced to Essential Oils I thought, "What a scam!" However I soon learned that not only did these essential oils do exactly what they promised to, but that using essential oils added a layer of support to my wellness practice. I learned that essential oils were a safer alternative for my family to support our lifestyle. Essential oils have been used for thousands of years, and we're still learning about all of the properties they have to offer. The number of clinical research studies incorporating essential oils keeps growing globally each year, and they are getting more mainstream acknowledgement which may be why you are here. In this book we will be exploring the basic properties of essential oils, the ways to use essential oils, the basic chemistry components and how they can be used in regards to blending essential oils together, and what simple ways you can use oils in your everyday life. I will be sharing my personal blending tools, focusing in on the fundamentals of essential oil safety, and how to use an essential oil routine to support your well-being to give relief to emotional and physical symptoms.

Essential oils are not DRUGS, however some oils can interact with medications you may be taking and so it's always important to keep your pharmacist informed of any new supplements or essential oils you are using.

WHAT ARE ESSENTIAL OILS?

Essential oils are just concentrated compounds that have been either pressed or distilled from plants. We'll be focusing in on the Monoterpene hydrocarbons, Sesquiterpenes, Phenols, Monoterpene alcohols and Sesquiterpene alcohols, Aldehydes, Ketones, Esters, Lactones, Ethers and Oxides. One of the newest forms of distillation that we'll discuss is Supercritical Fluid.

As a founding member of the IAC I started my life coaching business in the early 2000's. I found that helping others is my love language and the core of my soul purpose in life. Through my practice I have been able to live that dream and helps thousands of people every year.

For the last several decades I have worked primarily as an online holistic lifestyle and wellness coach. Working so much with essential oils I became a Certified Aromatherapist, although I am also a nutritional therapist. I work with families, niche market entrepreneurs and small business owners to create a holistic alignment for their ultimate success. With this book I am here to guide you in your own personal alignment using plants as joy, plants as support and plants as grounding. Your creation of a totally realistic lifestyle change starts right here with this book.

My Mission Statement is: Inspiring a nation of holistic beings to THRIVE as organically, functional authentic East Meets West Nourished Warriors living a 360 degree vibration based lifestyle. What that really means is that I want you to read through this book and have ideas and thoughts pop up that make your life better. I want you to start to look at nature as something powerful, and then maybe we will all start taking better care of it. I want you to realize that we need medicine, but we need plants. Once we only relied on the botanical sources of nature for our wellbeing, and now we rely only on the grocery store and Amazon. This is the time to create something more balanced and so we start with the simplicity of aroma.

I became involved with Essential oils when my daughter was very young, and she was given a routine of daily steroids for her asthma. What I found was that these steroids were stunting her growth. Through connecting to the wellness community and a pivotal moment of education from Robyn Openshaw, I removed dairy from her diet and removed her daily steroid use in a matter of six weeks. I turned to aromatherapy as a new way to help us purify the air in our house and the first time she asked for it herself, that is when I knew it was working. This change moved my coaching practice into a whole new world of wellness through plants, which was so aligned with everything else I was moving into in my personal life.

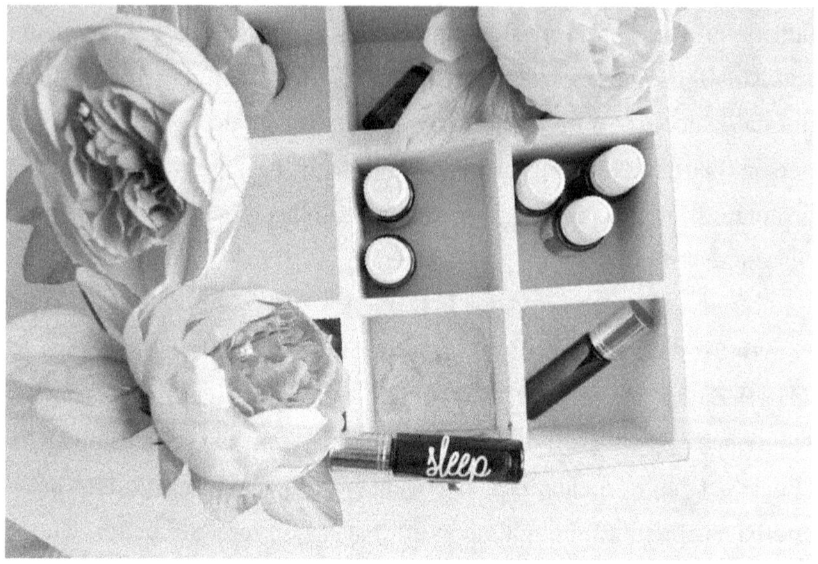

When we inhale a fragrance, the odor molecules travel up the nose where they are trapped by olfactory membranes, well protected by the lining inside the nose. Here the aroma will float to the back of the nasal cavity. Each odor molecule fits like a little puzzle piece into specific receptor cells lining a membrane known as the olfactory epithelium or olfactory membrane. This olfactory membrane is a layer of cells on the roof of the nasal cavity. Olfactory receptor cells are the only neurons in the nervous system that are regularly replaced, lasting only about four to eight weeks.

Our olfactory membrane is three layers of cells: the supporting cells, the olfactory receptor cells, and the basal cells. The supporting cells function as metabolic and physical support for the olfactory cells, which are actually neurons. The basal cells are stem cells and are the source for new receptors capable of division. These Basal cells can differentiate into either supporting or olfactory cells. But those neurons, which are called the Brush cells, are what respond to odors with an electrical impulse that is directed to the olfactory bulb.

Your olfactory bulb has sensory receptors which are actually a part of the brain that send messages directly to our lizard brain, the most primitive brain centers; where it influences emotions and memories, as well as where the "higher" centers modify our conscious thought. This amazing brain center perceives odors and then accesses your memories to remind us about people, places, or events associated with these olfactory sensations. This is the most powerful of our five senses and 10,000 times more sensitive than any other of the senses you have. Aroma gives us an immediate reaction. Because of the immediate connection we have to odors within our limbic system, it's easy to see that aromatherapy can impact memory and mood as well as behavior.

The structures of this complex limbic system are responsible for so much. The release of different neurotransmitters like endorphins and promoting the production and release of various neurotransmitters which impact the nervous system happen in the limbic system. Recent research has been done using learned odors with mice that gives us even more insight into what is happening in our body when we inhale. Using mice under anesthesia, as well as with studies using conscious sheep, researchers have been able to see an increase in the release of both glutamate and GABA in the olfactory bulb in response to these learned odors.

Glutamate and GABA are the brain's most plentiful neurotransmitters. Over half of all of your brain synapses use glutamate, and 30-40% use GABA. These two neurotransmitters have a complex and interconnected relationship and they have such a huge impact on so many different areas of our mental, physical and spiritual wellness that we need to address this connection. Glutamate is the excited neuron, where GABA is the relaxing neuron. Our GI tract is packed with GABA receptors, and supports the healthy levels of antibodies that protect our gut and mucous linings from harm. In fact there are more neurons in your gut than in the nervous system, and your gut brain is the main source for receiving information, processing information outwards, so that our body can react.

The body's emotional state within the "head brain" is mirrored in the "gut brain". We know for a fact that our gut is a huge center for our immune system, and all of those emotional substances psychiatrists think of when looking at the mental and emotional problems within the brain. Over ninety percent of our serotonin is created in the gut, and so this offers you a glimpse of how important it is to know what you are doing when you are using essential oils and how much we still need to research in regards to essential oils, nutrition and our bodies. If an essential oil can impact your brain it will impact your gut, and if it can impact your gut it will impact your brain. Knowing if we are creating an impact that is good or bad is why essential oil education has to happen on a broader scale than it has in the past.

With essential oils available at any store within a five mile radius in most town centers, we have to start talking about them more often than we are. People are becoming more educated with the growing number of essential oil companies, but there is no book that is required to start using aromatherapy, and there should be. Because you have to understand weight, dilution, storage, interactions in order to be an essential oil truth seeker. You wouldn't buy a bottle of medication and just start using with your child without understanding what it was, how it is used, and what the dangers are. So it should be with these oils.

When we talk about the weight of an essential oil, what we are really talking about is their scent characteristics. When you are blending single oils, it becomes a full bodied blend when you have a nice combination of top, middle and base note essential oil choices. Essential oils fall naturally into three groups. The most highly volatile essential oils, known as top notes in the perfume industry, are those that evaporate most quickly. These oils tend to have an uplifting and invigorating action. These are the fastest acting essences for the body.

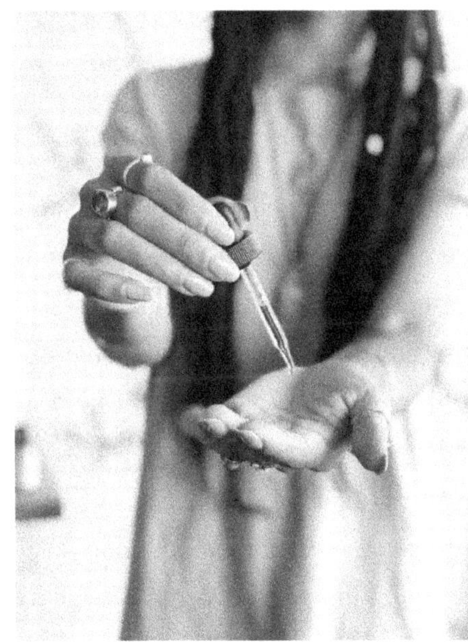

Essential oils that have slower volatility, will evaporate more slowly, and are known in the perfume industry as base notes. These oils are most often used therapeutically for their calming and sedating action. Essential oils with a medium range of volatility, known as middle notes in perfumery, act to stimulate and regulate. These base and middle notes are used when calming and relaxation is most needed.

Top Notes contain the smallest molecules and are the quickest to evaporate and are the first noticeable impression in a blend. These light oils like the citrus oils are often a scent that reminds us of spring, and these oils will move quickly from the aroma to a sharp tone, and do not last long aromatically. Citrus oils like Lime, Lemon, Mandarin, Tangerine, Grapefruit, Orange as well as Cinnamon, Eucalyptus, Clary Sage, Peppermint, Spearmint, Thyme and Tea Tree or Melaleuca are all considered top notes. Top notes aromatically evaporate within one to two hours.

Middle notes are those fuller, richer notes that really provide the heart and soul to your blend. They are soft, yet full bodied. Cardamom, True Lavender, Pine, Rosemary, Myrtle, Juniper, Geranium, Chamomile, Cypress, Marjoram, Fennel, Nutmeg and Ylang Ylang. These are the core oils of subtle changes and yet are often not a first choice because they are misunderstood, and because we like broad odors. Middle notes aromatically evaporate within two to four hours.

Base Notes are those deep grounding essential oils that will last the longest both in aroma and in storage when stored properly. Good quality Frankincense oils can last for two decades when stored properly in a dark, glass bottle in a cool storage area. Base note oils are the glue to your blend and hold everything together. My favorite base notes are Cedarwood, Sandalwood, Frankincense, Patchouli, Rose, Vetiver, Neroli, Myrrh, Jasmine, Ginger, Clove and Vanilla! Base notes usually aromatically evaporate in five hours, but may even linger for days being detected by your olfactory system. Where we love Top Notes because of the quick uplifting emotional connection, we love Base Notes because of the quick grounding emotional connection. Yet the best blends will offer a bridge from the top to the base, to balance the aroma energies.

Essential oils have been around for thousands of years. These volatile oils give plants their distinctive smells, and offer protection to plants, as well as play a role in plant pollination. In addition to their intrinsic benefits to plants and their beautiful fragrance, the components of essential oils have long been used for food preparation, beauty treatment, and health-care practices. I like to think of essential oils as holistic because they offer support to the whole body just as they do to the whole plant.

Egyptians were some of the first users or essential oils that we have recorded. They used aromatic botanicals when preparing the bodies of the deceased for burial. Some of the oils used were Cinnamon, resins like Frankincense and Myrrh, Spikenard, and early forms of Cedarwood and Juniper essential oils. Egyptians thought unpleasant smells were associated with impurity, and good smells indicated the presence of the sacred. They used three different forms of aromatherapy: burning, cooking with oils in animal fats, and combining oils for topical use. The word perfume literally means, through smoke, because of this ancient method of aroma fragrance. They blended their botanical plants with the oils from moringa and lotus, to create a conditioning balm. The funeral furniture of King Tut displays the pharaoh's wife wrapping his body with the lotus oil. These tombs also often contained "perfume" bottles. It has been documented that the ancient Egyptians used at least 21 different types of vegetable oils for cosmetic purposes, which I find completely fascinating. They took these oils and create a holistic approach to both wellness, and beauty.

WHAT IS HOLISTIC HEALTH AND BEAUTY?

Holistic (or Wholistic) Health is based on health as a whole or holism. All parts of the person make up the total health. Wellness begins with the whole rather than just a symptom. This includes organs, cells, body symptoms, and even emotions and what is going on in our environment. Holistic Beauty treats the inner and outer systems, personality, and emotional wellness in a holistic health manner to create a successful beauty treatments and beauty routine that is beneficial to the client's whole being to attain their beauty goal. The most regarded beauty brands and ambassadors in the industry are using holism in their products and services because it is so much more beneficial. Beauty brands with long waiting lists that incorporate energy healing alongside aromatherapy, meridian work and nutrition are the fastest growing areas in the beauty industry outside of influence based makeup brands.

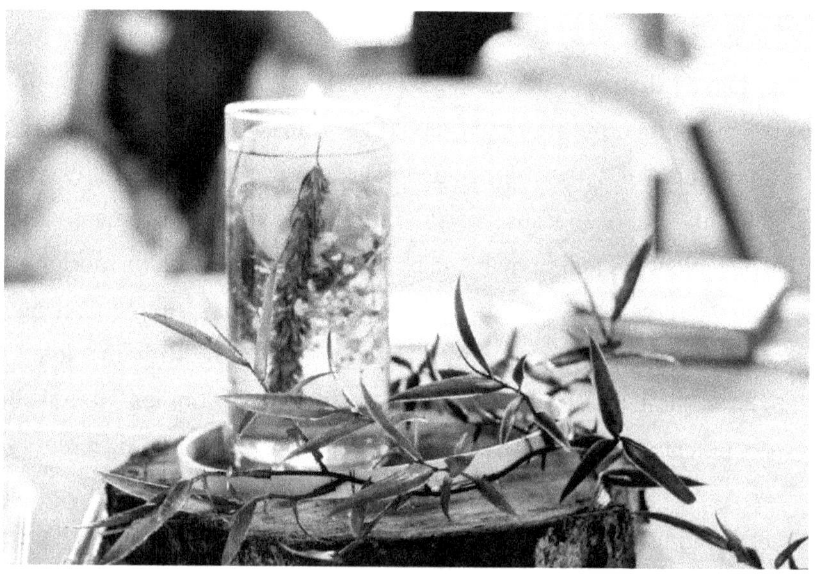

Essential oils offer multi-therapeutic functions in a holistic format. They offer both inner and outer system benefits, as well as giving a client the simple properties to address emotional needs at a bioelectrical level on their own. Looking at the entire person offers a better expectation of reaching a goal through the practice of holism-based therapies. Creating a beauty treatment or an aromatic blend is more than just dropping a few drops into a topical solution or diffuser. The total holism must be defined by the expectations of the client, and understand what their individual definition of beauty or wellness is. As well the goal must quantify the total beauty wellness vision to achieve that goal, and the methods of use.

Your total being has an effect on your overall beauty and the appearance of your skin. It is rare you will meet a person with an unhealthy inside and a glowing outside. We are what we eat, as much as what we put on our bodies. Biologically, and psychologically, the chemical toxins we come into contact with, the foods we eat, the way we treat our body through exercise and stress management are all going to have impacts on the skin. The skin is the largest organ of the body, and a very important part of the elimination process.

What is going on inside of your body can be seen by looking at your skin. The ability of your primary chimneys to repair and protect your body must be addressed in order to keep from over-eliminating from our skin. When you hear the saying, "Beauty is skin deep." it is true because deep in our cellular levels of our skin's makeup we can see the stressors, disease, and experiences of your daily life.

There are four primary toxin removal systems that must all be working in harmony with each other for healthy detox. These involve:

1. The disposal of cellular waste products, especially lactic acid.
2. The removal of larger waste products through your lymph (smaller waste products go into your veins and are exhaled or sent directly to your liver).

3. The processing of toxins by your liver, most of which then go into bile and then into your digestive tract for final clearance (some water-soluble toxins go to your kidneys to be excreted in urine).

4. The final clearance of waste products by your digestive tract.

These four systems tend to flow from one to another. Any glitch in any one of these major systems of detoxification will back trash up in your body and cause problems.

Your lymphatic system works directly with the cardiovascular system to help flush toxins out of the body. It also carries immune cells throughout the body to help defend against infections. But your lymphatic system isn't lucky enough to have some powerful organ like the heart to keep fluid flowing. The lymph system is stimulated by gravity, muscle contraction (exercise), hydrotherapy (alternating hot and cold water on the skin), breathing, lymph drainage therapy and massage. This is why we consider exercise to be such an important part of being holistically healthy.

If liver, kidneys and lungs do not fulfill their tasks sufficiently, the body needs help from the skin. The skin is the largest organ of protection and defense. Other types of waste products within the body, and chemical toxins are excreted in the form of rashes. Very few essential oils have specific skin regenerative properties, and so unless topically applying to the feet, I rarely apply any essential oils to my body without dilution. If someone tells you that your essential oil rash is just detox, please consider working with a different oil distributor. Although the body will create a rash from an overloaded system failure, it also will create a rash from improperly diluted oils.

USING AROMA IS ALREADY HAPPENING

When the flowers are blooming and the bunnies are jumping, this new season calls for opening the windows and getting outdoors. We want to smell these aromas, but there are also ways that aromatherapy can support transition in every season. When we look at how aromatherapy can be supportive to our bodies during the changing season, it is similar to seeing how the smell of a fresh rain storm or a field of flowers can have on your mindset. I know that we have all experienced the power of aroma—the smell of a flower reminding you of a summer at Grandma's house, or the smell of baking that reminds you of a trip to France. There is a science to aroma. Many oils offer this re-established balance and peace within our body when we are dealing with the transition of a season.

As I said before when talking about the olfactory bulb, sense of smell is one of our most important senses—and essential for our reptilian brain. It affects our behaviors, memories, moods, emotions, and even relieves those seasonal allergy symptoms. As well one drop can be both stimulating and calming, and essential oils offer that natural support. Essential oils are aromatic, and naturally occurring compounds that interact with each other in various ways - not just in balancing out top notes and base notes. When these oils are extracted from the flowers, roots, stems, bark, seeds and other parts of a particular plant, they synergistically can elevate the spirit and soothe the mind because of both chemistry and the limbic brain within. Through massage, direct inhalation, and diffusion, essential oils can balance and ground you.

Dust, smoke, animal dander, grass, flowers, trees and weed pollen impact us more than we would like to consider, so isn't it ironic that these same flowers can provide a natural, soothing solution. Essential oils have been scientifically proven to contain anti-inflammatory properties and support our bodies just like a natural antihistamine. As an example, since oils can have a direct impact on our limbic system, arousing the sensory stimuli offers an interesting support system during times of seasonal discomfort to promote clear breathing and overall respiratory health. Have you ever bought a menthol rub? That is a commercial example of an aromatherapy technique.

As an industry, aromatherapy is growing rapidly in both the retail sector and the medical research arena. We are starting to learn that as advanced as we are, this may be the time to step backwards. Growing evidence of superbugs, and even looking at how medical devices are working in our bodies, are making the world take notice that sometimes simple is the better answer. Beyond the simplest understanding of holism; what you eat, your activity level, environmental factors, and emotional health; we now know all of these play a part in our gene expression.

Gene expression is the new vogue as DNA companies are launching faster than we can keep up with them. Recently geneticists have been surprised to find that epigenetic change could be passed down from parent to child, one generation after the next, including all of these areas that impact our own gene expression. I love this quote by Dan Hurley, "The genome has long been known as the blueprint of life, but the epigenome is life's Etch A Sketch: Shake it hard enough and you can wipe clean the family curse." Nutritional epigenetics is interested in the way in which food affects patterns of gene regulation. Environmentally one of the biggest things I have seen talked about over recent years, is how many toxins can be passed down through generations. All of these areas can impact your DNA, and your children and grandchildren's DNA. This is all the science of epigenetics. Epigenetics, simplified, is the study of biological mechanisms that will switch genes on and off.

So how does this correlate to the use of aromatherapy in this new area of exploration? Essential oils can support your body as you work to find balance, and help to switch on or off genes to make our lives better just like we have seen in the latest nutritional research. In a recent study, the scientists conducted RNA sequencing using essential oils. RNA sequencing is increasingly the method of choice for researchers studying our cells. They used this RNAseq on over 30 different essential oils to see how each essential oil impacts the epigenetics of the human genome. What they concluded was that essential oils might influence many areas including growth and rejuvenation of particular types of cells.

So beyond gene expression, another way we are impacted by essential oils was written about in a book called, The Heart Code, written by Paul Pearsall. In this book he talks about the process by which essential oils actually unlock cellular memory, as it activates certain parts of the brain in the limbic system. Remember that the structures of the limbic system are responsible for the release of different neurotransmitters, and to promote the production and release of various neurotransmitters which impact the nervous system. Research has been done where they have seen the release of both glutamate and GABA; Glutamate is the principal excitatory neurotransmitter in brain, in that olfactory bulb in response to learned odors. The limbic system is where a lot of emotional baggage and emotions are stored. This increase in the oxygen to the limbic system actually helps the brain unlock the DNA and allows a lot of emotional baggage to be released from the cellular memory… which is what I love most about aromatherapy in today's world.

Pure essential oils will contain a vast amount of therapeutic constituents that your body can "pick and choose" from in order to rebalance its physiological processes. They not only possess general properties based on their biochemical makeup, but as you see, factors such as our own genetic variances, microbiota diversity, and "internal environment" all influence their actions.

The three rules for use of essentials oils are:

1) Look for transparency in quality of product. If a company isn't releasing their tests, or are showing up as synthetic in 3rd party testing again and again. It's probably not a great oil to use. The quote is, "the soil is in the oil" and it's true. Just like you want to buy foods that haven't been sprayed with toxins, you do not want any oil that has been in contact with any toxins along its journey.

2) Do not use essential oils internally without working with a certified professional. Most of the historical problems with internal use of essential oils has come from synthetics, or using far more than one drop. However, the canaries, those people that have especially strong reactions to most anything, can have a reaction to your natural and pure essential oil. This may stem from their nervous system interacting with their own epigenetics (such as genetic variances in detoxification enzymes), or having functional issues within their immune system. Regardless, it's always best to go very slow with essential oils, and start with aromatherapy using just a couple drops in your diffuser. It doesn't take much.

3) Pricing often showcases quality. Any $0.99 Frankincense is definitely not pure 100% Frankincense oil. If a company has been in business for three or four decades, they may have contracts in place to offer a great quality Frankincense at an affordable price point. However, that is rare. Stop shopping for your oils in dollar stores, and start looking to your Certified Aromatherapist in choosing your essential oils.

With the understanding that essential oils have this broad impact on your body, and your mind, when you are working on your own, find a company that gets their oils from the best sources for each plant, and that has hands on production work at the farms and fields where the plants and trees are being grown. It may be hard to understand but good soil is a rare commodity and not every plant can be grown in just any climate. A company needs to be engaged in every step of the process, from finding the best farms, to distillation, and testing. Did you know that essential oil extracts are often washed with alkali to improve the odor and taste and to hide the fact that poor solvents were used rather than top quality distilling? That is why it matter if your oil is being tested for purity, and if you have access to those tests. A bad essential oil will impact your genome as much as a good oil, but in very different ways.

Many oil labels now have batch numbers that you can use online to check on the testing behind the oil. Be careful of oils that have the words fragrance oil or perfume on the oil label, or that use the term nature identical oil as an indication of being a diluted blend. Some oils are concentrated or folded for use in making household cleaners, soaps, candles and other aromatic items. Folding an essential oil like Bergamot allows a company to remove the photosensitive chemicals so that it can be used in a daytime facial serum. So the Bergamot in your favorite serum is not the same properties as the Bergamot in your bottle of aroma oil.

Essential oils may be rectified or redistilled, which means they have been put through distillation once or more times to remove impurities. This can also be called re-distilled. This process is done to the essential oil, and not to the plant. Re-distilled oils are reheated after the steam distillation.

Fractional essential oils are few, and Ylang Ylang is considered a fractional distillation oil, as is camphor. What this means is that Ylang Ylang essential oil has five levels or grades of oil to select, from Extra to Complete. Each level or grade of Ylang Ylang is based on the amount of time that the plant has spent in distillation. Ylang Ylang Complete has more Sesquiterpenes and a richer aroma. It spends about fifteen hours in distillation. Ylang Ylang Extra is the first level of distillation and only takes about two hours. This is done as the timing of distillation of the plant base, unlike the re-distillation process. Camphor is also fractional and is referred to as white camphor, brown camphor, yellow camphor and blue camphor. White camphor is the light fraction that is most often used therapeutically.

Essential oils should be stored in dark-colored glass bottles to protect the oils from deterioration.

The global essential oil market is expected to reach USD $11.67 billion by 2022, according to a new report by Grand View Research, Inc. Growing consumer awareness regarding the wellness benefits associated with natural and nontoxic personal care products is expected to remain a key driving factor for global essential oil market over the forecast period. Europe is the leading regional market demand share exceeding 40% of the global use of essential oils.

What's the top essential oil being used today? Orange oil is the leading product segment and accounted for 29.1% of total market volume in 2014. It is an environmental friendly oil, which has made it suitable for use in place of toxic fragrances in beauty products and household cleaners. Orange oil is also used as a biological pest control agent.

If you have ever rubbed the skin of an orange, and smelled that gorgeous smell on your fingers, that is the aroma we are talking about. Orange essential oil is extracted from the fruit peel. This oil, when used in aromatically, is generous for lifting your mood, but is also can support your immune system, is considered to be very purifying, and has amazing cleansing properties. Just one single essential oil, you will find, can have a variety of uses. They can be high in antioxidants, or high in a chemical property that with one drop can offer a refreshing boost to your overall day.

Make sure you use only pure, tested oils from transparent companies. Start small and use just a few drops in a diffuser, always diluting when using topically with just one drop. Always work with a Certified Aromatherapist when deciding how to proceed beyond aromatherapy to beauty blends and internal use.

Essential oils are created from plants, and just like food they can be toxically loaded with chemicals. They are not witchcraft, and help in many ways for beauty, emotional support, and may even change your gene expression for generations to come.

2

EXPLORING HISTORY

We have talked a little bit about how essential oils were used in Egypt. So let's delve into the many ways that essential oils have been used throughout history.

The Herbal Classic of Shen Nong is an ancient Chinese medical text, listing 365 substances with their descriptions and medicinal uses. Shen Nong, also called the Divine Farmer, is the legendary originator of all Chinese herbal medicine. Many artifacts have been found in the same time period and region (Shaanxi Province, Western Zhou Dynasty) that would have been used for preparing and storing liquids, like those made from herbs. In addition to Shen Nong, Huang-ti, the Yellow Emperor, also included herbal medicine in his book on disease called —The Yellow Emperor's Classic Of Internal Medicine. There is so much that was written about in these ancient Chinese texts that we are just starting to figure out. The Yellow Emperor's Classic Of Internal Medicine is an ancient text on health and disease. This medical text has been treated as the fundamental doctrinal source for Chinese medicine for more than two millennia. These two texts hold many uses for aromatics that are still used by practitioners of traditional Chinese Medicine.

Shen Nong had three classifications for herbs, similar to the notes we have for oils: Upper, Middle and Lower. The nature of the drugs in the upper class is quite capable of expelling illnesses. The nature of the drugs in the middle class is more closely connected with curing of illnesses; one mentions them less frequently in connection with the liberation of the body from its material weight. The nature of the drugs of the lower class is especially suited for attacking a disease. The grouping of the herbs into three categories has been criticized, similarly to some of the discussions I have seen on notes, and where some oils have been classified in various notes.

The Ebers Papyrus was discovered in Egypt. Though this text is full of incantations and foul applications meant to turn away disease-causing demons, it also includes 877 prescriptions. This text may contain the earliest documented awareness of cancerous tumors. One of those prescription suggested cooking herbs and fruit in oil, and anointing it to "remedy the bowels." Similar to some of the ways we have used essential oils in my home over the last decade. There have also been other documents found that recorded the medicinal use of herbs in Egypt dating back to the days of the Great Pyramid being built, and the ancient Egyptian god Nefertem, was the god of perfume and healing.

The earliest known Greek physician practiced around 1200 BC combining the use of herbs and surgery. Hippocrates was the first physician to dismiss the Egyptian belief that illness was caused by supernatural forces. His treatments would typically employ mild physio-therapies, baths, massage with infusions, or the internal use of herbs such as fennel, parsley, hypericum or valerian. Hippocrates is said to have studied and documented over 200 different herbs during his lifetime. He often recommended fumigation, including "fumigation from below" as a therapy for gynecological disorders.

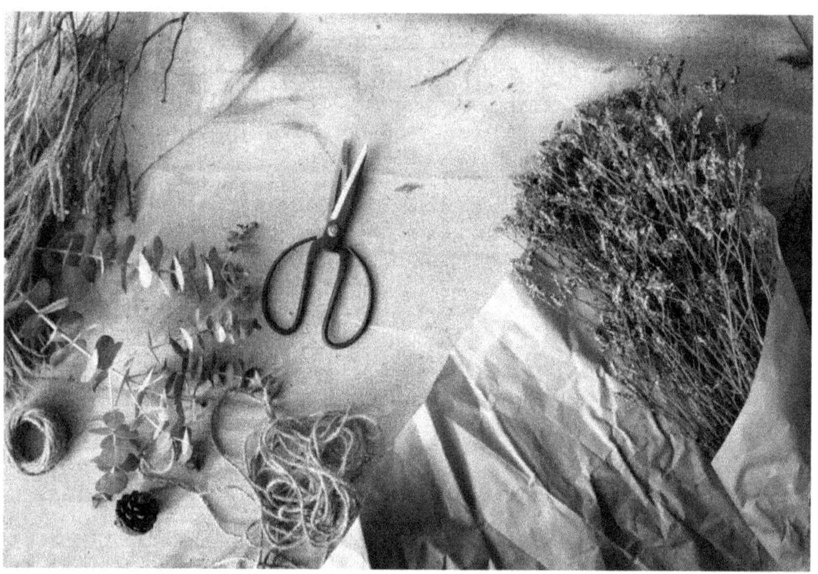

After Alexander's invasion of Egypt in the 3rd century BC, the use of aromatics, herbs and perfumes became much more popular in Greece prompting great interest in all things fragrant. Dioscorides, a military physician, traveled with the Roman armies to Greece, Germany, Italy and Spain, recording everything that he discovered. He described the plants habitat, how each should be prepared and stored, and described full accounts of their healing properties. His results were published in a comprehensive five volume work called 'De Materia Medica', also known as 'Herbarius'. He wrote about the medicinal properties of everything from almonds to aloes, aniseed, chamomile, cardamom, cinnamon, coriander, ginger, juniper, lavender, olive oil, peppermint, thyme and many more. In fact this volume contained 1000 different botanical medications, plus descriptions and illustrations of approximately 600 different plants and aromatics.

However the Greek doctor, Claudius Galen, was responsible for the first major classification of plant medicines into groups. Galen wrote many textbooks that were still in use throughout Europe during the Middle Ages and well into the 17th Century. His influence was so great that many historians use him as a sort of historical separator; Before Galen (meaning before Rome), and After Galen (meaning the Middle Ages and after). He prescribed French lavender as an antidote to poisons, and for uterine disorders. He is also often brought up in cannabis circles.

In his text called, "On the Properties of Foodstuffs" he says, "Hemp seeds are used to create a sort of warmth and/or given to party guests to promote hilarity and enjoyment. Others translations also add; "Hemp cakes, if eaten in moderation, produced a feeling of well-being but, taken to excess, they led to intoxication, dehydration and impotence." Galen also wrote about how Hippocrates fumigated the epidemic atmosphere at Athens during the plagues. Galen had his own fumigation process he called, Galene. This was where one would take in the drug by breathing, or swallowing, which he compared to the cleansing fire of Hippocrates fumigation. This may have been like modern incense, like the Kyphi, which was compounded incense from Egypt that was meant to be inhaled as an aromatic.

Galen's Cold Cream is a recipe invented by Claudius Galen in the 9th century. It makes a firm set cream which liquidizes almost immediately on contact with the skin. It can be used as a cleansing cream, hand cream or as an alternative to oil for certain types of massage. It was made with almond oil, beeswax, rosewater and drops of rose essential oil. You can find the recipe online if you want to make this ancient recipe for yourself.

One of the most talked about essential oils is created after the story of the Thieves. Of course as we talk about these "essential oils" it is important to remember that steam distillation of essential oils was invented by the Persian chemist Ibn Sina in the early 11th century. So most of what we have discussed as oils, were very crude compared to what we use today. However in the 15th Century, as the great plague was decimating Europe, four thieves were captured in Marseilles, France, and charged with robbing the dead and dying victims of the plague. This legend says although they spent their days robbing sick and dying people, they managed to escape contracting the plague and other similar awful diseases.

When the thieves were tried in court, the magistrate offered leniency if they would reveal how they resisted contracting the plague. They told of a certain potion of aromatic herbs, including 50 cloves and rosemary, and they rubbed it on their hands, ears and temples. The secret of the thieves was made public and the formula was posted around the city. I think it's important to note that the original Thieves essential oil was vinegar and consists of a variety of aromatic herbs. These included Clove, Cinnamon and Rosemary, as well as Eucalyptus and Lemon. I have seen many clinical studies showcasing how apple cider vinegar has multiple antimicrobial properties, and so there is no way to say if this story is true, what was the main secret to their staying healthy.

A German surgeon, alchemist and botanist wrote several books on essential oil distillation which went through hundreds of editions in every European language. In it he referenced 25 essential oils included rosemary, lavender, clove, myrrh. He was popular for his ability to both treat gunshot wounds, and for the creation of his distillation techniques. Distillation of essential oils is actually credited to the Persians, who invented the refrigerated coil in the distillation process of plants and made it possible to distill essential oils and floral waters (hydrosols). Alchemy is a philosophical and proto scientific tradition practiced throughout Europe, Africa and Asia. It aimed to purify, mature, and perfect certain objects, or to make something of little use, into something of great use.

During the 1600 and 1700's, a gradual decline in natural plant healing methods started as chemical medicines appeared One such chemical medicine was mercury. Although mercury did seem to cure syphilis, the neurologic side effects of mercury, were quite disturbing.

The role of microorganisms in disease was recognized in the 1880's and by 1887 French physicians first recorded laboratory tests on the antibacterial properties of essential oils. These early tests resulted from the observation that there was a low incidence of tuberculosis in the flower growing districts in southern France. In 1888 a similar paper was published showing the micro-organisms of glandular and yellow fever were easily killed by active properties of oregano, angelica and geranium. I still look to France for guidance in my own aroma practice.

In the 1980s, which was a very good decade, there was a Dutch Government report published that showed a women's skin is more permeable to toxic chemicals than men's skin. I find this so fascinating because women are the carriers of the next generation. The female skin is more permeable to essential oils, not because essential oils are toxic, but because oils are skin-permeable. This only applies to undiluted oils – as soon as they are mixed with a carrier oil, which is the way they are used in topical aromatherapy, the difference between men and women no longer applies.

Because skin absorption capability varies from one person to another, dilution is not only a safe practice, but an important practice. A woman's skin might still absorb better when essential oils are used with water, as in compresses or baths, but if there is a difference, it is only a small one, and not really worth changing up your topical application. You can to be careful about adding essential oils into your bath, remember that essential oils also work both percutaneously, not just through airborne inhalation. Percutaneous exposure is generally a much higher concentration.

Essential oil use has been around, and flourishing for thousands of year, and in modern times we are just beginning to grasp the opportunities. 'Aromatherapy' is one of the most actively growing forms of alternative medicine combining massage together with counselling and a nice odor. Most clients suffer from some kind of stress-related disorder and aromatherapy encourages the healing process largely through relaxation and the relief of stress. Stress is also a major problem in hospitals, hospices and homes for the aged and physically or mentally-challenged. Aromatherapy is welcomed by nurses who want to be closer to their patient and doctors who can refer patients with stress-related disorders who do not respond to conventional medicines.

The actual mode of action of essential oils in vivo is still far from known, although there is strong in vitro evidence that many essential oils can act as an antimicrobial or antioxidant agent or have a pharmacological effect on various tissues. Studies have shown that essential oils have an effect on brainwaves and can also alter behavior. It is possible that most of the effect of the oils is probably transmitted through the brain via the olfactory system. Used professionally and safely, aromatherapy can be of great benefit as an adjunct to conventional medicine or used simply as an alternative.

3

OLFACTORY SYSTEM

What is this Olfactory System? The olfactory system includes all physical organs or cells relating to, or contributing to, the sense of smell. When we inhale through the nose, airborne molecules interact with the olfactory organs and, almost immediately, the brain. This is accomplished by hydrocarbon and oxygenated compounds crossing the blood brain barrier. These molecules inhaled through the nose or mouths are also carried to the lungs and interact with the respiratory system. Thus, inhaled essential oils can affect the body through several systems and pathways.

Directly under the small match-head-sized bulbs is the cribriform plate, made of thin bone. The olfactory neurons pass through this plate and end in protein-rich cilia, inside the top of the nose. Here the receptor cells and ion channels convert an odor, and eventually into an electrical impulse to the brain. At the roof of the internal nose cilia are embedded in a thin layer of moist mucous about the size of two shirt buttons, on the top and either side of the nasal cavity. Into this mucous, project very tiny hairs. This forms the tip of the rod-like olfactory nerve cells, and there are between six and twelve hairs to each cell. The hairs are unprotected extensions of the actual neural cells, so that olfaction is exceptional among the senses in that it involves an extremely direct interaction between the neuron and the source of stimulation. The other end of each neuron leads directly to the olfactory bulb in the brain. Aroma molecules must pass through this before reaching the receptor cells on the cilia.

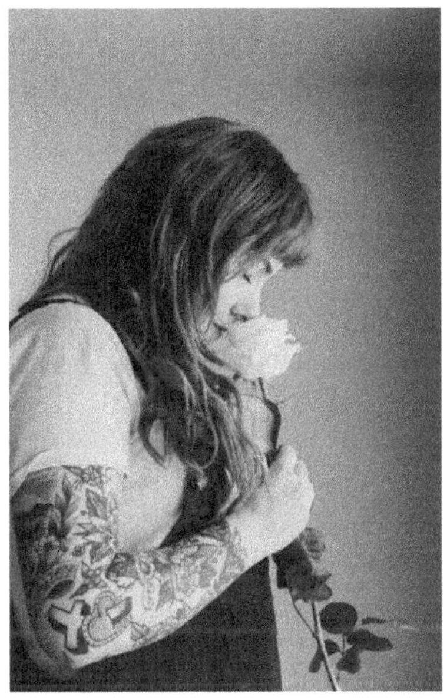

Take a smell in … Air movement is necessary for continued olfaction to take place. This is because the odoriferous molecules have a very short period of time for use, and have to be replaced by fresh ones. One thing that seems to take place with some odors is when the same odor is inhaled for more than a few seconds, the smell begins to fade, and may disappear entirely. Have a pet? This effect is far more pronounced with some scents than others.

When inhaled through the nose, certain aromatic molecules of essential oils enter the lungs from where they diffuse across tiny air sacs into the surrounding blood capillaries and eventually find their way into the systemic circulation from where they exert their therapeutic effect. Others travel to the brain.

However, it all starts with the olfactory bulb. This essential part of the olfactory system starts the process when odorant molecules enter our nasal cavity through inhalation or by rising from the mouth (e.g. during the chewing of food). It is an interesting part of our central nervous system, and the bulb is attached to the cerebral hemisphere by a long stalk often referred to as the olfactory stalk. The central olfactory system receives the odor molecule information through the axons of our sensory neurons.

This information is processed and integrated as the olfactory quality of objects. The human perception of the olfactory image is characteristic in that it usually associates with pleasant or unpleasant emotions. Studies of adults suffering from anxiety disorders have shown that they also possess enlarged, highly connected amygdalae. The olfactory system is the only sensory system that involves the amygdala and the limbic system in its primary processing pathway.

Rather than visiting the thalamic relay station on its journey into the brain, smell information travels directly to our olfactory bulb – with nothing in between. The thalamus is a structure in the limbic system, at the center of each cerebral hemisphere and is a relay for sensory pathways, and for brain stem, cerebellar, and subcortical pathways to our cortex. The thalamus also serves as a relay between cortical structures. The limbic system is comprised of the thalamus, hypothalamus, pituitary and pineal glands; and the stimulation of the hypothalamus and pituitary glands causes reactions in the autonomic nervous system and the endocrine system. What normally happens when you see, hear, touch, or taste something? That sensory information heads first to your brain's relay station. Then it sends that information to the relevant brain areas including the hippocampus, which is responsible for memory, and the amygdala, which does the emotional processing. The olfactory bulb is directly connected to our amygdala and hippocampus, which may be why the smell of something quickly triggers a detailed memory or even intense emotion response.

The olfactory epithelium, called the OE, is a specialized epithelial tissue inside of our nasal cavity. Epithelium (/ˌɛpɪˈθiːliəm/) is one of the four basic types of animal tissue, along with connective tissue, muscle tissue and nervous tissue. Epithelial tissues line the outer surfaces of our organs and blood vessels throughout the body, as well as the inner surfaces of cavities in many internal organs, like our nose. In mice, the OE contains more than 2 million sensory neurons, can you imagine? In 1991, Richard Axel and Linda Buck published a ground breaking paper that shed light on olfactory receptors and how the brain interprets smell. They received the Nobel Prize in Physiology or Medicine 2004 for this research. What they identified was a family of 7-transmembrane domain receptors, which are thought to be the first known olfaction receptors.

This was big news, and the summary of that research was that a large gene family, comprised of some 1,000 different genes (which are about three percent of our genes) that regenerate throughout our lifetime and that give rise to an equivalent number of olfactory receptor types. These receptors are located on the olfactory receptor cells, which occupy a small area in the upper part of that nasal epithelium that we just talked about. These receptors detect those inhaled odorant molecules. Each olfactory receptor cell possesses only one type of odorant receptor, and each receptor can detect a limited number of odorant substances. Our olfactory receptor cells are therefore highly specialized for a few odors.

The cells send thin nerve processes directly to distinct micro domains in the olfactory bulb. Receptor cells carrying the same type of receptor send their nerve processes to the same glomerulus. From these micro domains in the olfactory bulb the information is relayed further to other parts of the brain, where the information from several olfactory receptors is combined, forming a pattern. Therefore, we can consciously experience the smell of a lilac flower in the spring and recall this olfactory memory at other times.

It's because of all of this that essential oils are a valuable tool in unlocking emotions via olfaction. Once the odor molecules stimulate olfactory cells, the result is a nerve impulse that enters the brain via the limbic system. The hypothalamus is the message station for transmitting aroma messages to other areas of the brain. Oxytocin, the cuddle or love hormone is produced primarily in the hypothalamus. This is why a scent can turn you on or turn you off.

MEMORIES

Because the olfactory bulb is part of the brain's limbic system, an area so closely associated with memory and feeling it's sometimes called the "emotional brain". Clinical research has showed us that any traumatic experiences are stored on a cellular level and have profound effects on one's emotions and the physical state of the body. We can use aromatherapy to help us regain that balanced energies in our body and open our subconscious mind. Through my practice I have seen aroma help promote a sense of wellbeing, promote emotional release of negative stored memories, all through this penetration of the olfactory, and overall limbic system.

When you inhale the aroma, it also penetrates the hippocampus, where the storage of working memory and short-term memories take up residence. This is also where the pineal gland is, an area that has been associated with our spiritual development. Our sense of smell becomes mature at an early stage of development. Our sense of smell begins developing, as those olfactory epithelial cells form during our fetal development in the early pregnancy weeks along with the nostrils. These cells connect to molecules that bind with the olfactory nerve (which leads to the brain). After a baby develops a sense of smell, it can actually smell everything that you eat or inhale. Everything.

So where are those memories stored? In November 2017, scientists discovered that our memories may be saved in a part of the olfactory bulb itself. The part responsible is a complex structure called the piriform cortex. It is the largest and most distinctive olfactory cortical area. This new research leads us to believe that it would be more useful to regard the olfactory bulb as the primary olfactory cortex (primary in the sense that it is the first stop), while the piriform cortex should be regarded as an association cortex — meaning that it integrates sensory information with 'higher-order' information like our cognitive, contextual, and behavioral information.

In the European Journal of Neuroscience, and older study experimented with extracellular activity in response to odor. Cell activity was largely synchronized with breathing and different temporal patterns were observed. The anterior piriform cortex was characterized by odor-evoked responses phase-locked with the inhalation-exhalation transition period. So does breathing have something to do with these memories, or release of memories?

If we go back to Traditional Chinese Medicine, the Lung Meridian is responsible for the intake of energy in the body, just like it's responsible for the air we need to get oxygen... which as you know now is atoms of energy. This meridian is very connected to our Olfactory bulb and organs, and so I just see aromatherapy as a fantastic way to help rebalance the flow of energy, and seemingly to rebalancing memories, or perhaps letting them go. As an energy healer and Aromatherapist I see the lungs a carrier to bring in the energy from the essential oils, and distribute it to wherever it needs to go.

Now that we have discovered all of this information about the olfactory system, more and more research is happening. Associate Professor Dr. Stefan H Fuss has also has been doing research showing that the olfactory sensory neurons and taste cells are the only nerve cells in direct physical contact with the environment, rendering them vulnerable to environmental insult. His research shows that our nose is a remarkably sensitive system able to detect environmental chemicals in trace amounts and to discriminate among structurally very similar molecules.

The discriminatory power of the olfactory sensory system depends largely on the specificity of chemosensory receptor cells in the nose and their proper connection to the brain. Each individual olfactory sensory neuron expresses only one allele of a single olfactory receptor (OR) gene from a much larger genomic repertoire. This is where the structure of epigenetics can come into play, and how using chemically altered essential oils may be more damaging than we think.

What happens when the olfactory system has captured these smells and memories? Working with its limbic system it affects a wide range of behaviors including emotions and motivation, not just memory" (Athabasca University - Advance Biological Psychology Tutorials). It can impact instinctive or automatic behaviors, and shows little, if anything, to do with conscious thought or will. It is also translates the sensory data from the neo-cortex (which is our thinking brain) into motivational forces for behavior. This can be involved in the mediation between your recognition of an event, your perception of it as stressful, and the resulting physiological reaction to it, mediated via the endocrine system. You can see why the practice of (w)holism is so important.

Olfactory nerve cells are the only type of nerve cell in the body which can be replaced if damaged. Because of the high absorption of essential oils by the mucous membranes of the respiratory tract, they can be inhaled as airborne particles. The state of acidity in the delicate mucous membranes allows them to be very effectively absorbed materials into the body. The nose has many surface capillaries, through which molecules can go straight into the bloodstream.

When you first smell a new scent, you link it to an event, a person, a thing or even a moment. Your brain forges a link between the smell and a memory. Burnt gunpowder can trigger PTSD in a veteran, and in fact one way they are using aromatherapy is in introducing that trigger smell in a therapeutic safe space, so that the individual can feel safer when they experience the smell again.

How powerful really, is our sense of smell? Researchers at the University of California at Berkeley have found that humans actually have sophisticated olfactory capabilities. A group of 32 volunteers were asked to track scents with their noses across a 10-meter (about 33-foot) trail. The subjects were blindfolded and wore gloves and earplugs to isolate their senses of smell. Two-thirds of the volunteers were able to track the scent and, although they were slower than the tracking dogs, most improved with practice [source: BBC].

Most of the essential oil molecules you will inhale during aromatherapy will be breathed back out, although some will enter the bloodstream via the lungs and circulate through the body. Only eight molecules of an odoriferous substance are needed to trigger the smell mechanism. When specific odors are used with intention, the connection and experience are stored in our brain and remembered. When the odor is smelled again, it evokes an amazing response. The more an odor is used, the stronger the connection becomes.

What about the blood-brain barrier? The walls of the tiny capillaries that carry blood around the brain are very selective. Although tiny nutrient and oxygen molecules, and occasionally items like heavy metals can pass through the capillary walls, larger molecules, including most therapeutic drugs, and blood cannot. Aromatherapy by-passes this and goes straight to the brain through the olfactory system. The essential oil itself goes no further than the inside of the nose, but it triggers off a nerve impulse, amplified along the way, which has far-reaching repercussions.

In aromatherapy you may hear someone say that the plant or the oil knows where it is needed. David Stewart, Ph.D.,R.A. has explained that in the past we thought that the interstitial tissues of the brain served as a barrier to keep damaging substances from reaching our delicate neurons and the cerebrospinal fluid. More accurately, it is more like a sieve or filter, which only molecules of a certain size or smaller can pass. He said, "Doctors don't know for sure, but it seems that in order to cross the blood-brain barrier, only molecules less than 800-1000 atomic mass units (amu) in molecular weight can get through. Lipid solubility seems to be another factor which facilitates passing through the blood-brain barrier. Water soluble molecules don't usually penetrate into brain tissue, even when very small. The molecules of essential oils are all not only small, but lipid soluble as well."

When we look at those small essential oil molecules they are less than 500 amu, and that is why they are so aromatic, for our olfactory use. Certain Sesquiterpene constituents found in essential oils have been shows in research to directly cross this barrier because of this small molecular size. Monoterpenes are structurally smaller than Sesquiterpenes, which leads us to belief that they can also penetrate into the brain.

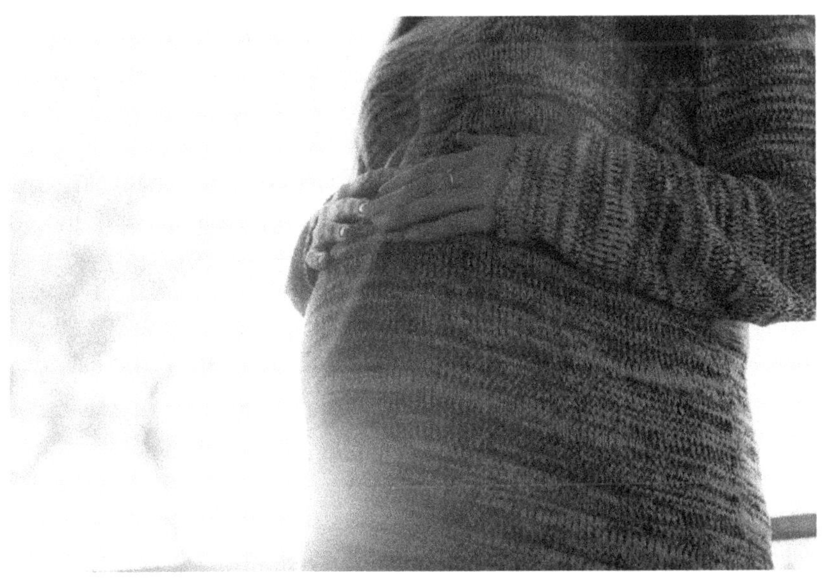

Our brains are very sensitive to environmental toxins, and one reason is that just a minute amount of neurotoxins, chemicals that can damage our brains, can impact us from the womb and beyond. Just like our brain has this wonderful limbic system, it also doesn't have this barrier before birth, and during those first developing years. Your brain doesn't regenerate easily, you're your red blood cells or your skin, and by 18 months of age newborn neurons migrate long distances to the olfactory bulb and the prefrontal cortex. This migration occurs in both streams postnatally, but declines steeply after 18 months of age and has almost completely disappeared by early adulthood.

Pacific salmon navigate towards spawning grounds, which we have seen here in the Pacific Northwest every year, using olfactory cues they imprinted on as juveniles. When we first moved here is was a favorite homeschooling field trip to see the return of the salmon, or visiting the salmon locks to see them swimming upstream so determined from the Puget Sound into the lake. The timing at which imprinting occurs has been studied extensively, and there is strong evidence that salmon imprint on their natal water during the parr-smolt transformation. This is the series of physiological changes where juvenile salmonid fish adapt from living in fresh water to living in seawater. Our sense of smell starts developing between 6 weeks and 7 weeks of pregnancy. All functional layers of the olfactory bulb are mature by the 22-weeks stage in your baby. That means that what you smell your infant smells, and their bodies are so much smaller than ours that you can understand why it's so important to be very careful of what essential oils you use while pregnant.

As well, the amniotic fluid is the first food of infants, and contains a wide range of nutrients that have particular tastes, such as glucose, fructose, lactic acid, fatty acids, and amino acids, as well as the flavors (for which the odors are perceived retronasally) of the foods consumed by the mother. Like essential oils can cross the brain barrier, so can those toxins. Some neurotoxins like lead, alcohol, and organophosphates can impact the brain development. Fetal alcohol exposure results in smaller olfactory bulbs and impairments in odor discrimination that persist into adulthood. Scientific reports show that maternal exposure to lead can be transmitted to your grandchildren. Another study that was reported in Medicinal & Aromatic Plants in 2015 revealed that like other substances, essential oils can influence the way our genes express.

Thirty one essential oils were used in the study including: (Peppermint [*Mentha piperita*], Bergamot [*Citrus bergama*], Wintergreen [*Gaultheria procumbens*], Grapefruit [*Citrus x parasisi*], Basil [*Ocimum basilisum*], Rosemary [*Rosmarinus officinalis CT cineol*], Orange [*Citrus sinensis*], Tea Tree [*Melaleuca alternifolia*], Clove [*Syzygium aromaticum*], Lemon [*Citrus limon*], Balsam Fir [*Abies balsamea*], Birch [*Betula alba*], Chamomile [*Chamaemelum nobile*], Cinnamon [*Cinnamomum verum*], Cypress [*Cupressus sempervirens*], Eucalyptus Globulus [*Eucalyptus globulus*], Eucalyptus Radiata [*Eucalyptus radiate*], Frankincense [*Boswellia carteri*], Ginger [*Zingiber officinale*], Helichrysum [*Helichrysum italicum*], True Lavender [*Lavandula angustifolia*], Lemongrass [*Cymbopogon flexuosus*], Marjoram [*Origanum majorana*], Myrtle [*Myrtus communis*], Oregano [*Origanum compactum*], Sandalwood [*Santalum album*], Spruce [*Picea mariani*], Tangerine [*Citrus reticulate*], Thyme [*Thymus vulgaris*], Vetiver [*Vetiveria zizanoides*],

Ylang Ylang [*Cananga odoratac*]); and were procured through an organization that I have used a lot in my home and my practice.

During this study cells were treated with essential oils for a period of six hours. Following treatments, the cells were harvested and RNA was isolated for expression studies. RNA was prepped and underwent next-generation sequencing. RPKM values, which are a measurement of the genes, were determined and set relative to the untreated control samples. Each particular essential oil is composed of a unique compliment of constituents, and thus potentially varies in their effects on living cells. They made sure to determine a dose high enough to elicit a biological response, yet low enough to avoid the induction of cell death.

After they determined a general sense of transcripts differentially regulated among essential oil treated cells, the next step was to further investigate expression profiles for changes that are unique to particular oil or to a subset of essential oils. Transcription is the process by which the information in a strand of DNA is copied into a new molecule of messenger RNA (mRNA). DNA safely and stably stores genetic material in the nuclei of cells as a reference, or template. RNA-seq is a powerful method to determine mRNA expression levels in cells. The researcher was able to use this method to evaluate the way essential oils can influence our gene expression. Epigenetic processes, including DNA methylation and histone modification, are thought to influence gene expression chiefly at the level of transcription. We can now safely determine that there is more to it than we previously thought, and that knowledge of this should make choosing toxic-free essential oils one of the most important things you can do for yourself.

Olfactory nerves are like other nerves and organs in the body. We are energy, and they respond to electrical signals and impulses that form coded messages dispatched to various areas of the body. These impulses may be why diffusing some oils will increase the production of endorphins, neurotransmitters, and antibodies.

The sense of smell is the only one of the five senses directly linked to the limbic lobe of the brain, the emotional control center. Anxiety, depression, fear, anger, and joy all emanate from this region. This is why the scent of a special occasion can evoke memories and emotions before we are even consciously aware of it. Where smells are concerned, we react first and think later. Odor can also be one of our greatest enjoyments, bringing back memories and creating feelings of security, grounding, and well-being, not just the bad memories and emotions.

The limbic lobe (a group of brain structures that includes the hippocampus and amygdala that is located below the cerebral cortex) can also directly activate the hypothalamus, our master gland. The hypothalamus is one of the most important parts of the brain, acting as our hormonal control center. It releases chemical messengers that can affect everything from our sex drive to energy levels. The production of growth hormones, sex hormones, thyroid hormones, and neurotransmitters, like serotonin, are all governed by the hypothalamus.

Essential oils – through their odor and unique molecular structure – can directly stimulate both the limbic lobe and the hypothalamus. This can exert a profound effect on mind and body. So besides feeling good when you diffuse an aroma, you can also stimulate the production of hormones from the hypothalamus that can result in increased thyroid hormone (our energy hormone) and growth hormone (our youth and longevity hormone).

Dr. Alan Hirsch of the Smell and Taste Research Foundation in Chicago, and his team have carried out forty-six research studies including one involving 12,000 people which looked at the effect of olfaction on learning. Among other things, Dr. Hirsch has discovered that people will judge a product a better value when bought from a shop where there is a pleasant aroma. In another trial he found that when a mixed floral aroma was suffused throughout a room of calculus students, they increased their speed of learning by 23%. When gambling machines in Las Vegas were —aromatized with a certain aroma, Dr. Hirsch discovered that the players spent 45% more cash!

Dr. Joseph Ledoux, of the New York Medical University discovered that the amygdala plays a major role in storing and releasing emotional trauma. He found that using aroma may create a profound effect in triggering a response from this gland. He theorized that this could be a major breakthrough in helping to trigger the release of pent-up emotional trauma.

In studies conducted at Vienna and Berlin Universities, researchers found that Sesquiterpenes in the essential oils of Sandalwood and Frankincense can increase levels of oxygen in the brain by up to 28%. Such an increase in brain oxygen may lead to a heightened level of activity in the hypothalamus and limbic systems of the brain, which can have dramatic effects on emotions, learning, and attitude.

There are so many new research studies every day on the impact aroma can have on our bodies, our emotions and our energy. It's important to remember that olfaction is the most direct interface between the brain and the rest of our world.

When we inhale, the odor molecules travel up the nose where they are trapped by olfactory membranes well protected by the lining inside the nose, then floats to the back of the nasal cavity. Each odor molecule fits like a little puzzle piece into specific receptor cells lining a membrane known as the olfactory epithelium. The olfactory membranes are very tiny and well protected, and contain about 800 million nerve endings that receive the micro fine, vaporized oil particles, carry them along the axon of the nerve fibers, and connect them with the secondary neurons in the olfactory bulb. Each one of these hundreds of millions of nerve cells, these are replaced every 28 days.

This lining of nerve cells triggers enzyme activity and electrical impulses via the nerve pathways to the olfactory bulb, which then transmits the impulses electrical impulses to the olfactory bulb, which then transmits the impulses to the gustatory center (where the sensation of taste is perceived) the amygdala (where emotional memories are stored and is the memory center for fear and trauma), and other parts of the limbic system of the brain and the cerebral cortex and the olfactory sensory center at the base of the brain. These aroma molecules set off a cascade of reactions involving proteins, enzymes, cell depolarization, and second messengers – all leading to an electrical impulse being sent to the cerebral cortex and the limbic system. The part of the brain most directly involved is the limbic system, evolutionarily the oldest part of the brain, and home of our emotions. Nerve messages from our sense of smell travel faster to the brain than those from any of our other senses.

The message is received by the limbic system which is the seat of emotions and memory, and consists mainly of: the amygdala, which houses instinctual behavior, emotions, memories; the hypothalamus, which controls the autonomic nervous system, body temperature, hunger, and thirst; and the pituitary, which receives messages from the hypothalamus and sends chemical messengers into the blood, releasing hormones that regulate body functions. People who have undergone nose surgery or suffer olfactory impairment may find it difficult or impossible to detect a complete odor. The same is true of people who use makeup, perfume, cologne, hair sprays, hair coloring, perms, or other products with synthetic odors. These individuals may not derive the full physiological and emotional benefits of using essential oils and their fragrances, but we just don't know. Understanding the olfactory system better with time, we may found that the "smelling" is only a part of it.

4

AROMA CHEMISTRY

When you are delving into essential oil education, just understanding the basic chemistry can help you create better choices for blending oils together. What I want you to know is that this is a complex area, but if you learn a few key ideas, blending will become second nature.

What is an aroma? When we talk about aroma, we are talking about the thing that is perceptible to the olfactory sense of smell. Since as humans, we can differentiate between up to 10,000 different aromas, that's a lot going on in the olfactory system. Aromas, which are chemical compounds, bond, to form molecules. These chemical compounds have a smell or odor when they are sufficiently volatile to be transported to the olfactory system. Volatile just means that is has the tendency to vaporize. Essential oils are also often called, volatile oils, whereas aroma compounds are classified by structures. These are Esters, Linear Terpenes, Cyclic Terpenes, Aromatic, Amines (a-meen), Alcohols, Aldehydes, Ketones, Lactones, Thiols and a small variety of miscellaneous compounds. The known chemical constituents of plants are of two kinds: products of primary metabolism and products of secondary metabolism. The first are mainly carbohydrates, amino acids and fixed oils, produced by photosynthetic or their light-absorbing processes. The latter group of chemicals arises from the primary metabolites. They include the glycosides, terpenoids, alkaloids and essential oils. The chemical composition of DNA in plants and humans is virtually the same.

These plants that we get our essential oils from were the first life forms to appear on the land surface of our Earth. One of these first plants was conifers. Some of these types we recognize as evergreens have managed to survive to the present, even after flowering plants came to dominate the landscape several million years later. The bristlecone pines are the oldest plants we know of that we have, and redwoods are the tallest. Pines and other conifers were able to compete for water and ward off bacterial and insect invasions by evolving specialized ways. These plants had a way of moving fluids as well as manufacturing secondary metabolites.

What is a secondary metabolite? Secondary metabolites are not necessary for maintaining the life of a plant like chlorophyll containing cells are, however, they do contribute greatly to the quality of the life of a plant and help determine its long term survivability. They assist plants to fight off disease, live through a drought, defend against predators, heal their wounds, and communicate with others of their kind, facilitating interspecies communication, and reproduction. Essential oil molecules that were created by evergreen plants, as secondary metabolites many millennia ago are among the most ancient chemical constituents found in aromatherapy.

When we talk about chelation, people often think about supplements, and detoxification. Chelation is actually a type of bonding of ions and molecules to metal ions. While plants have antioxidative and DNA-protective components, like humans they also have a chelating component. This chelate is a chemical compound composed of the metal ion and the chelating agent. An example in our own bodies we have our heme part of hemoglobin, which is the substance inside red blood cells that binds to oxygen and sends the oxygen released from plants into the blood, as our chelating agent. Green tea extract can cross the blood brain barrier to attach to and remove excess iron that has stored in our brain, and that is what you may think of as iron chelation. What we are really talking about is similar in the idea of chelation being about bonding. Within a plant the similar agent is chlorophyll, which is responsible for the green color of plant leaves. Hemoglobin and Chlorophyll have very similar structures. The main difference is that chlorophyll is built around magnesium and our hemoglobin is built around iron as the central atom. Our bodies need hemoglobin to transport oxygen from the lungs to other parts of the body. How this happens is that the heme contains a chelating agent bonded to an iron ion.

With chlorophyll, the metal at the center of the chelate is that magnesium ion. Chlorophyll absorbs the light energy that is converted to chemical energy in the process of photosynthesis. So if we start to think about the way plants can work within the body, this is essential to understand that it is a chemical reaction, and as such, a lot of what we see in plants, are going to work similarly in our own bodies. I say this because if we look closer at chlorophyll, when ingested it can help do the job of hemoglobin. It can promote the health of circulation, cleanse the body, increase the number of red blood cells and therefore increase oxygen throughout the body by helping build hemoglobin. This similar chemical composition of plants and our bodies may explain why essential oils seem to act like keys to our physical and mental mechanisms.

Every cell in the body has its atoms lined up in such a way that it has a negative and a positive voltage, inside and outside. As energetic bodies we, like the rest of the universe, are just made up of mostly these components of energy. This is where that idea of the law of attraction is based in science. If you reach down right now and touch your arm, or the computer you are using; you can touch these items because of the fact that we are ultimately composed of atoms which are made up of interacting subatomic particles. If we could access an ability to control our bodies at this subatomic level, we could perhaps walk through walls because at this subatomic level we are all just energy.

Now we may call what we feel atoms, which is the basic unit of a chemical element. A strong chemical bond is formed from the transfer or sharing of electrons between atomic centers. Atoms tend to arrange themselves in the most stable patterns possible and this relies on the electrostatic attraction between the protons in nuclei and the electrons in the orbitals. The force that holds atoms together in collections known as molecules is referred to as a chemical bond. If the body is minute molecules, it's important to understand that a chemical bond is what is taking place. Generally, energy will be released when a bond forms between two atoms, no matter what type of bond.

Essential oils that we generally talk about, are composed of only volatile aromatic compounds, and must have a low molecular mass. Molecules cannot be collected by steam distillation if they have a molecular mass above the low 300s. Steam distillation is a special type of distillation (a separation process) for temperature sensitive materials like natural aromatic compounds. When talking about steam distillation, the steam passes through the organic matter that contains the compounds for separation. The steam condenses against that matter to form a mixture. Once the distillation is accomplished the vapors are condensed, there is the separation of the constituents at ease.

With CO_2 extraction we get some of those larger molecules that are unable to be steam distilled, and what you end up with is closer in chemical composition to the original plant from which it is derived, as it contains a wider range of the plant's constituents. The CO_2 Extraction of German Chamomile flowers yields a green extract, retaining less denatured oil. Pressurized carbon dioxide becomes liquid while remaining in a gaseous state, which means it, is now "supercritical." In this state it is pumped into a chamber filled with plant matter. Because of the liquid properties of the gas, the CO_2 functions as a solvent on the natural plant matter, pulling the oils and other substances such as pigment and resin from the plant matter. The essential oil content then dissolves into the liquid CO_2. At the end the CO_2 is brought back to natural pressure and evaporates back into its gaseous state, while what is left is the resulting oil.

A study using the Japanese Fern, and they found that when an oil was extracted using supercritical $C02$ Extraction, 27 compounds were extracted from the fern. With Steam Distillation, 45 compounds were extracted. However there were only 11 common components. So each oil has is place in aromatherapy, however the use of a Supercritical CO_2 extracted Turmeric, may be different than the use of a steam distilled Turmeric oil. It is important to understand the difference when looking at clinical studies or deciding on an oil to use for your personal practice.

Elements are substances consisting of one type of atom. Over 95 percent of the dry weight of a flowering plant is made up of three elements—carbon, hydrogen, and oxygen—taken from the air and water. It used to be believed that of the first 92 elements on the periodic table (1 is hydrogen and 92 is uranium) that 90 elements occur naturally. It is now believed that 98 elements can be found in nature. However you will only find five of these elements in your essential oil constituents. Among the macronutrients essential for a plant, phosphorus shows a great importance as an integral component of cells and as a respiratory and photosynthesis intermediate. However we know that the most common elements we are going to find are those carbon, hydrogen, and oxygen.

Essential oils are divided into three main groups based on the number of isoprene bonds they contain. An isoprene bond is a common organic compound. The MEP (methylerythritol phosphate) pathway provides a route to isoprenoid biosynthesis in the plastids of plants. While this sounds really complicated, the truth is that this is just the pathway by which the natural essence of these secondary metabolites are created via their own bio-factors. The cells of the plant have two different mechanisms to secrete their chemical classes including the Monoterpenoids, Sesquiterpenoids and Phenylpropanoids, Acids, Alcohols, Ketones, Aldehydes, and fatty acids and their Esters. In addition, those several nitrogen and sulfur compounds, impart characteristic sensory properties, which are also important constituents of many essential oils. Isoprene units can be linked either head to tail to form linear terpenes or in rings to form cyclic terpenes. Terpenes belong to a class of compounds known as Aromatic Hydrocarbons, and they are made up of those chains of linked isoprene units. Terpene Hydrocarbons are classified according to the number of isoprene units: Monoterpenes: 2 isoprene units, 10 carbon atoms. Sesquiterpenes: 3 isoprene units, 15 carbon atoms. Diterpenes: 4 isoprene units, 20 carbon atoms. Triterpenes: 6 isoprene units, 30 carbon atoms.

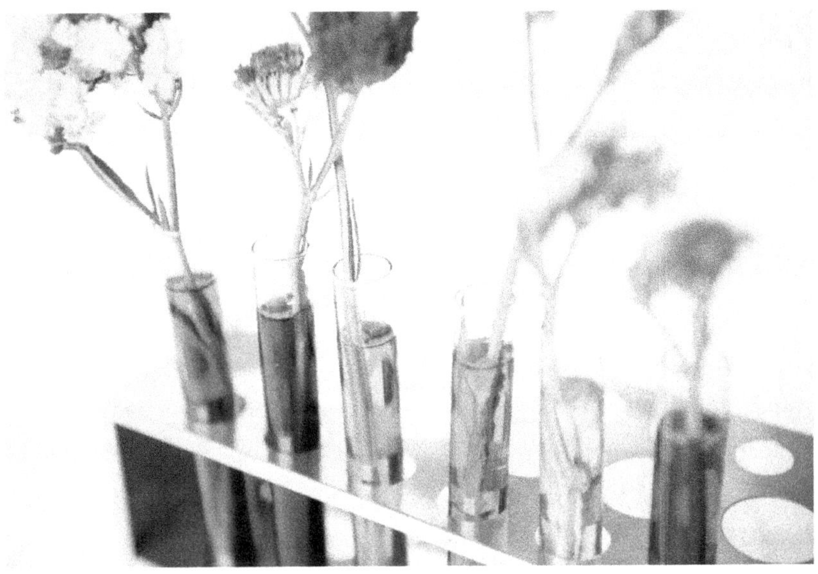

Carotenoids are a Tetraterpenes: 8 isoprene units, 40 carbon atoms. Beta-carotene in a carrot, it is a linear terpene that has 8 isoprene units, with 40 carbon atoms, whereas the Myrcene (pronounced meer-seen), specifically β-myrcene, is a monoterpene and the most common terpene produced by cannabis. Thus β-myrcene contains two isoprene units, and 10 carbon atoms. Isoprenes will absorb into our skin, fat cells, brain matter and the bloodstream rapidly permeating our bodies while bypassing normal digestive pathways. Again, this is the beauty of essential oils, and aromatherapy, and important to understand why essential oil safety must be a top priority.

Essential oil compounds belong to the Phenylpropenes which has one isoprene bond, the Monoterpenes which has two isoprene bonds or the Sesquiterpenes which has three isoprene bonds. These divisions make up those functional groups of essential oils. These include: Aldehydes, Ketones, Esters or Oxides, Lactones, Sesquiterpene Alcohols, Sesquiterpene Hydrocarbons, (pronounced fre-niel-proanes) Phenylproanes, Phenols, Monoterpene Alcohols, (pronounced fre-niel-propains) Phenylpropanes and Monoterpene Hydrocarbons.

Aldehydes, also referred to as Monoterpene Aldehydes, are often sweet smelling essential oils, who's formal, International Union of Pure and Applied Chemistry which we will call (IUPAC) from here on out, their IUPAC names always ending in —al Aldehydes are named with the suffix -al in order to designate the presence in the molecule of a carbonyl group. That means a carbon atom attached to an oxygen atom by via a double covalent bond and a single hydrogen atom - rather than a second chain of carbon atoms - attached to a carbon atom at the end of a chain of carbon atoms. The only exception is formaldehyde which is also known as methanol. It is the simplest of all the aldehydes in structure. When you think of aldehydes in essential oils you initially think of citral, geranial, neral, or even cinnamaldehyde. These oils are highly reactive, and so you must take care in use with aldehydes in aromatherapy. When you think of aldehydes you will often think about Lemon, Lemongrass, Melissa, Citronella and one of my favorites, Eucalyptus Citriodora. The aldehyde properties will vary from oil to oil, but you will often find oils supportive of helping with calming, inflammation, supporting healthy digestive and gi functions, and protecting against environmental threats.

Aldehydes are considered polar. Essential oils with oxygen-containing functional groups are polar at the oxygen atom site. These also include Alcohols, Phenols and Ketones. Oxygen is more electronegative than carbon, and so it pulls the electrons in the carbon-oxygen bond towards itself. This creates an electron deficiency at the carbon atom. Aldehydes are neutral liquids possessing a strong characteristic smell and are soluble in water. It is important to point out that as the carbon content of the molecule increases, they become less soluble in water, and their smell becomes less marked with the increase in boiling point.

Careful storage of essential oils high in Aldehydes is crucial. In studies done by UK-based scientists they claim that excess heating of some vegetable oils release high concentrations of Aldehydes, which can cause headaches, fatigue, and even dementia or worse. These Aldehydes can develop a not-so-great aroma when they have been overheated, or at the highest temperatures become odorless solids. Working with a company that knows how to properly extract your oils, and at low temperature is key.

Aldehydes often irritate the skin more than other essential oils. Take care to dilute these oils appropriately. Foundationally essential oil are either considered to be hydrophilic or wet/water soluble, or lipophilic or dry/oil or fat soluble. Aldehydes are classified in the wet oils. The more lipophilic molecules are absorbed quickly, but also vaporize more readily; the more hydrophilic components may be very slow in penetrating, if at all, but are also influenced by the presence or absence of occlusion, such as with compresses. Occlusive ingredients create a physical barrier helping to trap moisture in the skin or hair. The direct entry of lipophilic components from essential oils via the olfactory mucosa is quite substantial.

So there is a yin and a yang to consider as you select oil, and how best to work with it, and why I would rather not see anyone using essential oils in their bath water, especially with young children. Just don't do it. Later I will give you more detailed information on how to use essential oils in bathing. Dr. Kurt Schnaubelt, who has a PhD in Chemistry, wrote the book, "*The Healing Intelligence of Essential Oils:*, he talks clearly about essential oils being blended with Epsom salts rather than a carrier oil in order to promote the absorption of the essential oil rather than inhibit them in the bath. He also says, like Dr. Daniel Penoel has recommended, using a drop of an oil on a wet body in the shower offers an advantage to dilution and absorption into the lipophilic (fatty) skin tissues. However this is in discussion of using essential oils with adults, and not children. There are safety issues that parents do not think about before adding an essential oil into their baby's bath water. You may think that many baby shampoos have essential oils in them; however the high level of dilution is key.

Ketones may be identified from their IUPAC names always ending in "-one. This is a type of compound that contains a carbonyl group (C=O) that attaches itself without a hydrogen atom to a carbon on a chain structure, called an aliphatic ketone. So the oxygen atom is bonded to a carbon atom, which is itself bonded to two or more carbon atoms. Ketones are not very common in the majority of essential oils, and aromatic ones are particularly rare.

There are Monoterpene ketones, Sesquiterpene ketones and Diketones. Monoterpene Ketones are used often in skin care because they help support tissue and cell formation, however they can be very neurotoxic. Thujone is a neuroactive Monoterpene Ketone that is seen in Wormwood, Tansy, and common Sage. It is GABA receptor antagonist and excites the central nervous system. Ketones are molecules that we consider to not be "user friendly" to those that are sensitive to neurotoxic properties. So to administer them you must do so with knowledge and care, and know which oils should not be used with people who have Epilepsy. Ketone molecules are an irritant to the central nervous system and their general therapeutic effects are: strong mucolytic, promote skin regeneration, wound healing agent, as well as internally being potentially neurotoxic and hepatotoxic.

The oils we want to keep away from anyone that would be sensitive to these traits are Rosemary, Fennel, Sage, Eucalyptus, Hyssop, Camphor and Spike Lavender. I also will sometimes recommend not using Basil or Wintergreen depending on the actual use, and the client that is using the essential oils, and what their doctor recommends. In my practice I also stay away from others oils without a doctor's approval. Those oils include Basil, Birch, Coriander, Eucalyptus, Fennel, Oregano, Peppermint, Rosemary, Wintergreen, and any blend that contains one of these or other at risk oils, and in any products that may use these oils in their base ingredients.

A survey of the literature shows essential oils of eleven plants to be powerful convulsants (Eucalyptus, Fennel, Hyssop, Pennyroyal, Rosemary, Sage, Savin, Tansy, Thuja, Turpentine, and Wormwood) due to their content of highly reactive Monoterpene Ketones. You can find more information through PubMed at https://www.ncbi.nlm.nih.gov/pubmed/10460442.

Organic Facts lists that Mugwort's "soothing and the relaxing effects of this oil" makes it very calming unlike other Monoterpene Ketones we have discussed. That is why it is important to always look at the full chemistry of an essential oil before using it.

Carvone is a Monoterpene Ketone that has not been talked a lot about. A mouse thujone study was looked at for the treatment of diabetes mellitus; however a dose-related incidence of seizures was noted in 2-year National Toxicology Program studies in rats and mice. Now instead they are looking at carvone for regulating carbohydrate metabolism. I keep seeing other monoterpenes as well being looked at in pharma research studies, and so I think we will start seeing more of this type of clinical research in the future. Yet it is a good thing to see longer trials to make sure we have an understanding of what the risks are associated with the oil or compound being used.

Sesquiterpene Ketones and Diketones may how up in Cedarwood, Grapefruit and Helichrysum. There was a wonderful journal article that showed that there are fragrant Sesquiterpene Ketones as trace constituents in Frankincense volatile oil of Boswellia sacra. The largest and most widespread occurrence of the species is in northern Somalia. Diketones are the regenerative properties we've previously only found only in Helichrysum. Generally when you hear about Diketones, it is use in vaping, which is very different than the natural Diketones in Helichrysum, although I would still not vape any essential oils at all as this has no research studies on risks. Ketones are also considered to be more hydrophilic in nature.

Esters, also known are the most calming of the essential oil groups, and are some of my favorite essential oils. These oils result from the reaction of an alcohol with an acid and can be very most balancing of all the essential oil out there. I put the Esters with the Oxides because people often place them together in theory and in essential oil blends. Esters are more neutral where Oxides are more positively charged. Both Esters and Oxides are more lipophilic, though more balanced to also be closer to hydrophilic than those hydrocarbons are. I consider Esters to be the number one balancing oils.

Esters are a very important part of insect communication, and the alarm pheromone of the honeybee. Ethers are considered to be responsible for some of the hallucinogenic properties of certain essential oils when taken orally, so do not take these oils orally without working with a formally trained Aromatherapist. My favorite Ester is Clary Sage, which is so balancing.

Monoterpene Esters are often fruity and sedative in nature. These oils include Bergamot, Clary Sage, Roman Chamomile, and Lavender. The Phenylpropane Esters are also very harmonizing to our nervous system. Think of Basil, Tarragon and Fennel in this category. Phenylpropane Esters have a little more of a positive charge or polarity than Monoterpene Esters do, which gives them an ability to attract or acquire additional electrons. The only oils in this area that I really worry about people making sure to dilute very, very well are Birch and Wintergreen.

Oxides are more of the expectorants in this zone, and far more mentally stimulating. A favorite Oxide is Eucalyptus, although people don't realize there are a large variety of eucalyptus oils, as there are over 600 species of eucalyptus plants. The most common eucalyptus is Eucalyptus Globulus which is the one that I never recommend using on children, and yet is generally the most common oil people select. As well, Peppermint and Rosemary are also all avoided in younger children as all three of these essential oils have similar compounds. Most types of eucalyptus oils can cause central nervous system and breathing problems in young children, rather than helping respiratory problems. This oil should not be "applied to or near the faces of" or "otherwise inhaled by" children under 10 years of age. All of the soothing baby chest rubs have Eucalyptus Radiata in them, rather than Globulus.

You can make your own balm, or I love Maty's All Natural Baby Chest Rub. Coconut oil and beeswax are good to mix together and add a few drops of Eucalyptus Radiata. I love rubbing a blended balm on tiny feet or a little on the clothing but not on the chest with children. Always make sure to dilute your essential oils accordingly.

Peppermint, which is also very high in Esters, is often used to help reduce fevers. The problem with this is that it can cause an infant or toddler to go into shock due to the quick drop in temperature. Education is knowledge, and knowledge is power when it comes to using essential oils. Buying the large essential oil safety book is something I recommend to everyone if you plan on using essential oils in the future.

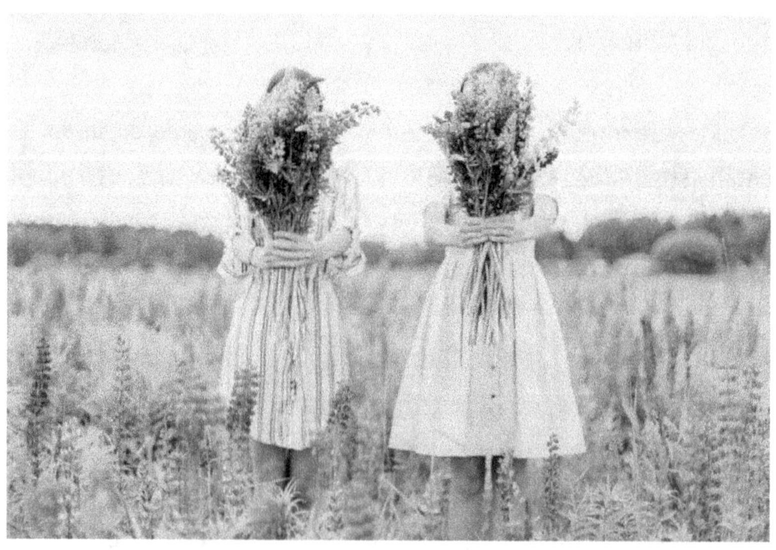

Popular oils that are considered to be Esters are Bergamot, Cardamom, Jasmine, True Lavender, Geranium, Clary Sage, Peppermint, Rosemary, Rose, Roman Chamomile, and Ylang Ylang.

Lactones & Coumarins are another great group of oils. These Lactones are a carbon ring with an ester attached. The Coumarins are a type or subgroup of these Lactones and have sedative effects. Lactones are like the diagonal opposite of Esters and are also very balanced. They are considered to be a special Ester, but they are a little more similar to ketones as they are principally closer to a Ketone than an Ester. I love Fennel, German Chamomile, Lemon and Lime. Lactones are found mostly in expressed and absolute essential oils.

I have always connected the Lactone oils with oils that release deeply stored emotions. One of the best oils is Patchouli, and as it ages the Lactone levels increase. In fact, as we will next discuss, when you look at the Monoterpene oils, they are mostly combined Esters and Lactones. Because Lactones are in a similar polarity and are also more water soluble and you will find they are therapeutic like those Ketones in oils like Fennel and True Lavender. One of my favorite Lactones is Sweet Inule from Corsica (which I learned about in my Milady textbook in Cosmetology school), and of course your cat's favorite Lactone is present in catnip.

The Coumarins are more green and grassy, and have that sort of an aroma. Those citrus oils like Bergamot that have a phototoxic warning, that component of the oil comes from being furanocoumarins which is a derivative of the subtype. Funny that they are green and grassy aromas, as several Lactones are considered germination inhibitors, and Coumarin is one of the most potent inhibitors known. You may find it interesting that Coumarin brings about an induced dormancy in non-dormant lettuce seeds. When the outer layer, or otherwise known as the flavado, of a half or a whole lemon or orange peel is removed and put into a big petri dish in which a small petri dish is placed containing 50 wheat grains so that there is no direct contact between them, the germination of the wheat grains is completely inhibited by the flavedo. Every have someone tell you that one drop of an essential oil is powerful? It is reasons like these that I find learning more about your essential oils can help you understand how and why they may be used, and why less can be all that you need.

Monoterpenes make up the largest amount of terpenes and can be subdivided into groups that indicate their structure. We are looking at both Monoterpene Alcohols and Monoterpene Hydrocarbons in this program. The Monoterpenes are often referred to as top notes for your blending purposes. These oils in general offer that stimulating effect, but they can also be skin-sensitizing if used for long periods. These classes of terpenes that consist of two isoprene units that have joined together head to tail and form the basis of all Monoterpenes, and the Monoterpene Hydrocarbons have at least 10 carbon atoms arranged in a chain.

Monoterpenes are found in many fruits, vegetables, and herbs. They prevent the carcinogenesis process at both the initiation and the promotion/progression stages. Oils with the suffix of -ene, refer to those Monoterpenes. Think about limonene or pinene. The Monoterpenes have several cellular and molecular activities that could potentially underlie their positive therapeutic index.

The monoterpenes inhibit the isoprenylation of small G proteins. Isoprenylation just refers to the addition of a hydrophobic isoprenoid group to a protein to facilitate attachment to cell membranes. Small

GTPases, also known as small G-proteins, are a family of hydrolase enzymes that can bind and hydrolyze GTP. There is a lot of talk in our aging process and ATP, but GTP is also a feature we look at in the Krebs Cycle. Listen to the keto podcasts and you will hear conversations about both of these.

ATP is used to carry energy for almost all energy-requiring chemical reactions in almost all cells. GTP can occasionally be used to carry energy, but it is more often used as a signaling molecule. One study done in May 1998 found that Monoterpenes have been shown to both prevent and treat mammary cancer in animal models and are currently in clinical testing in advanced cancer patients because of the inhibition of type I GGPTase. Not that you are going to cure anything with your essential oils, but it is interesting to know where the clinical approaches from essential oils are happening as they are looking deeper into the chemical properties.

Monoterpene Alcohols are more hydrophilic (remember meaning wet/water soluble) and the Monoterpene Hydrocarbons are more lipophilic or dry/oil or fat soluble. You may find that you want to use your Monoterpene Alcohols in your diffuser, and the Hydrocarbons mixed with carrier oils and applied topically, even though those Monoterpene Alcohols are generally tolerated topically. In France they would be applied to the wet body. You would get out of the shower; apply the oil which will be diluted by the water, and then step back into the shower to finish rinsing off.

The Monoterpene Alcohols are considered to be the safest of all of the aromatic oils. Tea Tree and Ylang Ylang are two of my favorites, and Geranium is great for skin care products. The Monoterpene Hydrocarbons are the most abundant in essential oils. Those wonderful needle trees and those citrus oils all contain monoterpene hydrocarbons. These can be skin irritating, which is why I recommend dilution with every lipophilic oil. Those include the Esters, Hydrocarbons and Oxides.

Frankincense is one of my favorite Monoterpene Hydrocarbon oils, as is Cypress. And if you have ever made pine needle tea, the Monoterpenes is what they consider to create the microbe-fighting action. My daughter was taught to make tea out of pine needles in her outdoor class this past year, and really loved it. Just add some untreated pine needles to a stainless steel pan full of boiling water and reduce the heat to simmer for about 15 to 20 minutes. Then pour it into a container and just let it sit overnight. In the morning strain out the pine needles, sweeten to taste, and enjoy your tea either by warming it up, or as a nice cold refreshment.

Sesquiterpenes was my favorite word to learn as I learned about essential oils. It's just fun to say. Sesquiterpenes are naturally occurring alcohols that very rarely exist in volatiles oils, meaning being able to evaporate at low temperatures. Because they are larger in structure, they have a greater potential for stereochemical diversity. Find an oil that has a stronger odor, and you are generally finding a Sesquiterpene. As terpenes, they oxidize over time into alcohols. Sesquiterpenes are found naturally in plants and in insects. They are the most diverse group of isoprenoids and in plants they function as the pheromones and juvenile hormones.

Approximately 5000 Sesquiterpenes have been recorded to date. Many fungi accumulate Sesquiterpenes. Some sesquiterpenoid Lactones are antimicrobial, disrupting the cell wall of fungi and invasive bacteria, whereas others protect the plant from environmental stresses that would otherwise cause oxidative damage. I find it interesting that algae is both high in those rich omega-3s and Sesquiterpenes. Both lettuce and chicory represent the main dietary sources of Sesquiterpene Lactones. These oils can have a longer half-life because they are less volatile. My favorite Sesquiterpenes are Cedarwood and Sandalwood. Cedarwood oil contains the highest amount of Sesquiterpenes. As an example the alcohol content of Texas Cedarwood oil ranges from 35-48%.

My favorite Cedarwood, Atlas Cedarwood, can be used in place of Sandalwood, and is much more affordable and much more sustainable. Until this year no sustainability program for Sandalwood existed in India. Australian Sandalwood has been regulated since the 1920s, with management of wild harvesting, and important to understand as sustainability is now a major challenge for many essential oil-bearing crops. Companies that are not looking at sustainability as a core focus, or that have been fined for importing oils from non-sustainable sources illegally, are ones you should stay away from. Atlas Cedarwood has a very low risk of extinction, but we should still make sure these are sustainably managed.

Sesquiterpenes have been promoted with the most benefits of any oil property I have found. Recently the hydrocarbon fraction of 30 virgin olive oils was analyzed, focusing in particular on the Sesquiterpenes. Just like Monoterpenes, Sesquiterpene Alcohols are more hydrophilic and the Sesquiterpene Hydrocarbons are more lipophilic or dry/oil or fat soluble. The Alcohols in skin care products are usually used in tonics, and the Hydrocarbons in anti-inflammatory oils. My favorite Sesquiterpene Hydrocarbons are Cape Chamomile and Myrrh.

When I think of Phenols, I think of Clove, Cinnamon and Oregano. My daughter would call these spicy oils, and these oils you HAVE to dilute no matter what. Phenols, sometimes called Phenolics, are a class of chemical compounds consisting of a hydroxyl group (-OH) bonded directly to an aromatic hydrocarbon group. These are defined by an alcohol function attached directly to a phenyl ring. Phenols have names which generally end in _ol' and there are only four common Phenols found in essential oils: thymol, carvacrol, eugenol, and chavicol. There are two Ethers from Phenols and the one is from eugenol and one from (pronounce chavicall) chavicol. Chavicol is an allylbenzene found in Bay Leaf and Betel Leaf, which is pepper and kava essential oils. As well, Spicy Basil is known as Methyl Chavicol. A lot of people may not know about Spicy Basil, but it is a much known oil in India and has been used in Ayurveda for centuries.

The essential oil of Oregano was one of several plant oils, when recently studied, that demonstrated protective effects for LDL against copper-induced oxidation. The most pronounced effect was observed with Oregano oil and the activity was attributed to carvacrol. Wilson's Disease is caused by mutations in the copper-transporter gene ATP7B, and for many people this is important because mitochondria are integral to metabolism and highly susceptible to damage from excess copper. They think this is caused by copper-induced disulfide bond (thiol) formation. According to Wikipedia Thiol is an organosulfur compound that contains a carbon-bonded sulfhydryl (R–SH) group. Thiols and alcohols have similar connectivity. Now phenols are not alcohols, and are far more acidic than alcohol. Thiophenols are these foul-smelling colorless liquids that are the simplest aromatic thiol. Phenols can be converted to the thiophenols. So now that may make more sense how Oregano could be helpful in this research area.

Phenylpropeneas the syllable '-en' in propene indicates the double bond, as opposed to phenylpropane. In certain plant families or genera Phenylpropanoid compounds are also found in the essential oil, sometimes as the main component.

There is not a lot of information that you will find in regards to Phenylpropeneas (pronounced Fre-neil-propanes) but they are very important in regards to an important plant specialized metabolic pathways called the phenylpropanoid pathway. Flavonoids are valuable natural products derived from the phenylpropanoid pathway. Phenylpropanoids have been found to have various pharmacological properties, such as antimicrobial, analgesic, anti-inflammatory, immunostimulatory, and expectorant activities (Kurkin, 2003). They also play important roles in plant physiology and defense by serving as pigments, phytoalexins, UV protectants, and insect repellents (Hahlbrock and Scheel, 1989). If we look at a vascular plant like basil or turmeric within the pathway once p-coumaric is activated by acid, this is the common precursor of these (pronounced Fre-neil-propanes) Phenylproanes, and the flavonoids.

These are considered to be Phenylpropanoids which has also been called Hemiterpenes. Some of my favorites in this area of course have the highest content, like Clove. I also love Cassia, Cinnamon, Basil and Oregano. I have read that these important Phenylpropanoids clean the receptor sites on the cells which is just amazing. While terpenes make up the largest single class of compounds, these Phenyl-propanes tend to have the largest impact on the aroma (Waterman 1993). Phenylpropane Ether which is found in Fennel, Tarragon, Basil and Aniseed can be toxic to the nervous system at high dosages. Here is another reason to keep your oils in a safe place and away from children or others that do not have the capacity to understand the dangers.

When you start looking at the properties associated with your essential oils, it is because of this relation to their chemical makeup. Some are very simple, and others very complex. No two oils are alike. Some constituents, such as Aldehydes found in Lavender and Chamomile, are antimicrobial and calming. Eugenol is antiseptic and stimulating. Ketones, also found in True Lavender, stimulate cell regeneration and liquefy mucus. Phenols are highly antimicrobial. Sesquiterpenes, predominant in Sandalwood and Frankincense, are soothing to inflamed tissue and produce profound effects on emotions and hormonal balance. Understanding the chemistry of an essential oil can help you determine how to best create a blend, or substitute when you do not have an oil a blend recipe has recommended.

Clary Sage should be used in moderation as it can have a psychotropic effect. Unfortunately, this creates an exaggerated drug-like state. It is important to warn anybody using Clary sage oil not to take alcohol, as it will produce dramatic if not unpleasant or colorful dreams. It is not normally used on those with cancers and estrogen-dependent tumors. This is because people with estrogen-dependent tumors (such as breast or ovarian cancer) should not use oils with estrogen like compounds, like clary-sage, as this can exacerbate the cancer. Therefore, I recommend it is safest not to use Clary Sage with any type of cancer. Women who are pregnant or trying to conceive also must not use it. Clary Sage should also not be taken in conjunction with other medicines or other substances that have an iron base.

Only use antimicrobial essential oils like Eucalyptus when necessary. Rotate antimicrobial essential oils rather than using the same oil again and again. Take caution in using Eucalyptus Globulus. Dilute well as it can cause a rash, itchiness, or irritation. Give a skin patch test before using this oil regularly. Hypersensitivity has been reported (Goodman & Gilman 1942, Lownefeld 1932, Schwartz and Peck 1946, Schewartz, Tulipan & Peck 1947). No irritation or sensitization at 10% dilution when tested on humans (Opdyke 1975d). Due to its internal toxicity, it should not be ingested as it can even be fatal from intestinal irritation in even minute doses. There have been many cases of Eucalyptus Globulus oil poisoning. Always make sure you work with a Certified Aromatherapist and doctor before taking any essential oil internally.

Eucalyptus should not be applied to the face, particularly the nose, and it can cause laryngospasm and as discussed it can cause over-excitement in babies and young children and most types of Eucalyptus are not recommended for use with children. Eucalyptus Radiata is the exception. You may use this oil in moderation for a few days at a time. Do not use during Eucalyptus while pregnant or trying to conceive.

Some homeopathic doctors believe that the scent of the oil negates the effect of homeopathic remedies and that using these two alternative therapies concurrently use should be avoided. Always check if someone is taking homeopathic remedies.

There are no phototoxic effects reported for distilled Lemon oil (Opdyke 1974i). The expressed Lemon essential oil is phototoxic (Opdyke 1974h). This will cause the skin to sunburn if exposed to the sun right after application; you should wait several hours keeping the skin covered before exposing skin to sunlight. In the case of expressed oils it is very important to ensure that the fruits have not been sprayed with chemicals.

Patch tests showed a barman, who complained of chronic eczematous lesions on the hands and occasional lip swelling and axillary itching, to be sensitive to Lemon, Lemongrass and Neroli essential oils and the component (jer-rain-eol) geraniol; sensitivity was attributed to (+)- limonene (structurally similar to geraniol) (Audicana & Bernaola 1994). Use this oil in moderation and only for a few days at any one time. Add only 3 drops at the most when using.

Lemon oil is a commonly adulterated essential oil. Terpene waste fractions left over from the industrial refining of citrus products and/or synthetic limonene is often purchased from chemical houses and used to dilute or "extend" genuine Lemon oil. Since terpenes and limonene naturally occur in lemon oil, even a gas chromatograph cannot distinguish between synthetic and natural limonene. Lemon essential oil can be cut with orange, distilled lemon oil, concentrated juice from vacuum extraction, synthetic limonene, citral, dipentene. BHA, BHT. Make sure that you purchase Lemon essential oil from a company that extensive testing beyond gas chromatography.

Occasionally, people may have allergic reactions to Tea Tree oil, ranging from mild contact dermatitis to severe blisters and rashes. Remember to use the skin patch test first. Again only use antimicrobial oils when needed. This oil is possibly sensitizing in some people. Undiluted Tea Tree oil may cause skin irritation, redness, blistering, and itching. There are many cases reported of skin irritation and dermatitis involving tea tree oil (Bhushan & Beck 1997,

Southwell, Freeman & Rubel 1997). This essential oil contains oxides and can negate the effects of an anesthetic.

Remember that Tea Tree oil is cultivated, grown from seed, and therefore the composition of the oil when distilled is variable. This oil is then adjusted at source to conform to laid down parameters and so may not have the natural synergy that may be expected. Tea tree oil has a relatively simple composition (about 30 compounds) and therefore is easily synthesized in the laboratory and this does happen all of the time. This is known as reconstructed oils (RCO) and is not a natural product and may have unwanted side-effects. Tea tree is often blended with other tea tree oils to attain standards settings. Tea Tree can be adulterated with other terpenes. Seven people had been applying commercial tea tree oil undiluted on the skin for conditions such as fungal infections, pimples and skin rashes and all developed eczematous dermatitis, some with vesiculation: a common allergen was (-)- limonene: application of diluted oil to the skin caused no reaction (Knight & Haussen 1994). Use of the commercial oil undiluted is ill advised.

Tea Tree may cause irritation to sensitive skins. Apply only a small amount when first using Tea Tree oil, and only after skin testing. Discontinue use if irritation appears. The oil should not be applied to non-fungal rashes or to broken skin. Do not use homeopathic remedies with Tea Tree essential oil as it can antidote them. The tea tree oil in commercial toothpastes and mouthwashes is generally considered to be acceptable because it is not swallowed. Avoid homemade tea tree oil mouthwashes. Several cases are reported of non-fatal poisoning where relatively large amounts of the oil have been ingested (Carson & Riley 1993, Jacobs & Hornfeldt 1994), Morris et al 2003). Application for chronic atopic dermatitis with undiluted Melaleuca was unsuccessful and then oral ingestion of the oil mixed with honey was advised, which led to exacerbation of the dermatitis. Don't use Tea Tree oil if you are pregnant or breastfeeding. Keep all Tea Tree oil out of the reach of children.

Care should be taken by those with sensitive skins when using Black Pepper essential oil. Although Black Pepper has been studied as being helpful using aromatherapy to help stop smoking, always use in the lowest concentrations topically as it may irritate the skin. Do not use during pregnancy. Do not use for a person who has high blood pressure. Black pepper is considered quite an irritant to the colon and liver is high doses. Do not use for a person who has a condition in the colon and liver.

Pink Pepper is also to be a concern for those with cashew nut allergies. It is commonly used in body care products and other beauty products, as well as a more recent popular essential oil. This oil could cause an anaphylactic reaction in someone allergic to cashew nuts or similar proteins.

Camphor should not be used by pregnant women. Camphor essential oil is one of my widely use oils for respiratory, in the most popular chest rub from around the globe. It is a 66–98 foot high tree, with a lifespan of 50 to 150 years. Camphor oil is not expensive, but it should be used wisely, and only when needed. The sustainability of camphor is affected by harvesting procedures. In Japan, the root, trunk, and branches of the tree are all used, whereas in the US, only the leaves and twigs of the oldest trees are used, thereby causing less injury to the tree. Only white, lightly filtrated, Camphor essential oil is used in aromatherapy. Brown, yellow and blue camphor oil are extremely toxic. When camphor oil is distilled only from the leaves, it is known as Ho-Leaf oil. Ho Wood and Ho Leaf oils are often used by compassionate therapists as a more sustainable substitute for the endangered Rosewood oil.

Do not use oil Grapefruit and Bergamot essential oils with a person who is taking pharmaceutical drugs, and use caution with Lime and Orange essential oils as there are possible interactions with those as well. Research shows that grapefruit juice blocks a special enzyme in the wall of the intestine that prevents many drugs from being absorbed into the body, making it easier for these medications to pass from the gut into the body, raising the blood levels of these drugs, which can create dangerous, toxic effects.

Peppermint essential oil may also cause an increase amount in the body of a calcium channel blocker that is used to treat high blood pressure levels.

Avoid Sage and Rosemary with high blood pressure medications as well. Avoid Angelica, Birch, Cinnamon, Clove, Balsam Fir, Helichrysum, Bay Laurel, Nutmeg, Oregano and Wintergreen when you are on blood thinners unless you are being monitored by your doctor.

When using antidepressants Clove (bud, leaf, and stem) and Nutmeg should be avoided due to possible blood pressure changes, tremors or confusion. Also consider avoiding Holy Basil, West Indian Bay, Cinnamon Leaf and Parsley Seed essential oils. Aniseed, Lemongrass, May Chang, Honey Myrtle and Lemon Myrtle should be avoided as the oil may potentiate drug action. German Chamomile, Yarrow, Blue Tansy, and some of the (art-tay-meese-uz) artemisias. These can affect the metabolism of Codeine, Lidocaine, (ama-trip-talean) Amitriptyline, Elavil, (imma-pra-mean) Imipramine, Tamoxifen, Prozac Paxil and other SSRIs.

If you are on Anti-diabetic medication avoid Lemongrass, and May Chang, Honey Myrtle and Lemon Myrtle should not be taken orally. These essential oils: Anise, Star Anise, Cassia, Cinnamon Bark, Dill, Fennel (bitter and sweet), Geranium, Lemongrass, May Chang, Melissa, Myrtle, Lemon Myrtle, Oregano, Savory and Turmeric, may influence blood sugar levels.

Some children with ADD/ADHD have (sa-lis-a-lates) salicylate sensitivity, aspirin sensitivity. Birch and Wintergreen contain methyl salicylate.

Anise, Star Anise, Cassia, Cinnamon Bark, Cinnamon Leaf, Clove (bud, stem, leaf) Cornmint, Fennel (bitter, sweet), Garlic, Lavandin, Marigold, Myrtle, Onion, Oregano, Patchouli, Ravensara Bark, Savory, Tarragon, Thyme have some inhibiting properties for platelet aggregation and may exacerbate the blood-thinning action of Warfarin or other blood thinners.

If you are on Methadone, Propofol or Tamoxifen do not use oils high in citral, such as Lemongrass, May Chang, Honey Myrtle, Lemon Myrtle, and Lemon scented Tea Tree oil. Rosemary, Eucalyptus, Ravintsara and Bay Laurel (Laurel Leaf) are contraindicated for those on barbiturates, as they induce rapid metabolism of these drugs.

Do not apply essential oils where you are or have been applying a transdermal skin patch. The oils may speed up or slow down the delivery of the drug, thus altering the dose.

When using H2 blockers or proton pump inhibitors and internal essential oils you are risking the enteric coated capsules to dissolve earlier in the stomach. This coating is used to prevent absorption in the stomach. Avoid all respiratory oils for a week prior to surgery.

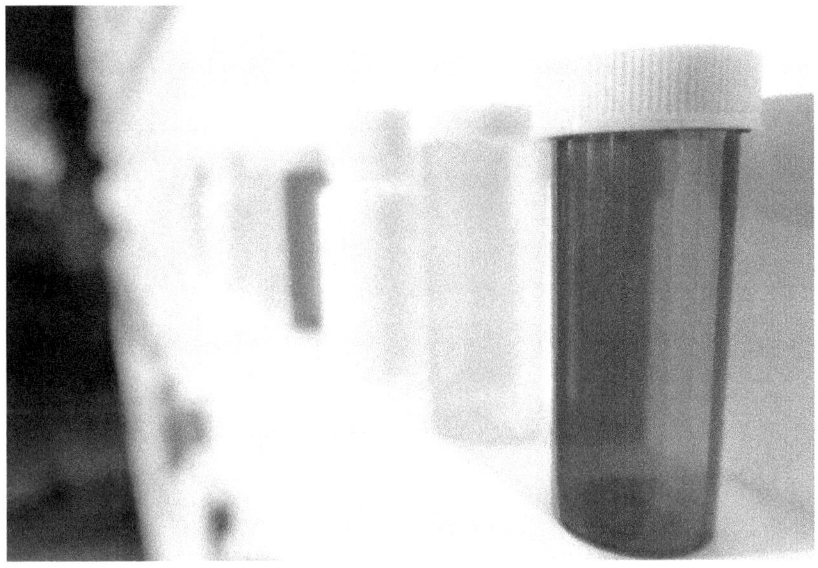

Always talk to your doctor and pharmacist about how your medications and alternative practices may interact with each other. This information is applicable ONLY for therapeutic quality essential oils. This information DOES NOT apply to essential oils that have not been assessed for quality, purity, and standardization of constituents. Remember that there is no quality control in the United States for essential oils and oils labeling. This information is for information purposes only and is not intended to diagnose, treat, or prescribe for any illness.

It is estimated that only 10% of the plant kingdom has been assessed for the essential oils they contain. With over 300 essential oil types being sold today, there is only going to be more possibilities for additional essential oils if we take care of the planet we have. As we have seen, synthetics are not going to give us what nature can. Take care of the planet and you will be the most important chain in the aromatherapy life cycle. Use essential oils safely, and you will benefit greatly.

6

BIOPHILIA HYPOTHESIS

Have you ever looked into a meadow, or rolled down the window and the aroma was just amazing. It seemed to pull you in and create another level of living. Biophilia hypothesis is the idea that humans possess an innate tendency to seek connections with nature and other forms of life. The term of biophilia was used by Erich Fromm, a German-born American psychoanalyst, in *The Anatomy of Human Destructiveness* in 1973 which described biophilia as "the passionate love of life and of all that is alive." This term was later used by American biologist Edward O. Wilson in his work Biophilia in 1984, which proposed that our tendency as humans was to focus on and to affiliate with nature and other life-forms has, in part, as a genetic basis.

Ethnobotany is everything we know as the power of plants. This of the plants used throughout history for medicine, food, fiber, dye, and more. For many of us the plants around us have become like a movie backdrop, and we have stopped focusing in on them. As we stop looking and listening to nature, sometimes we forget how much nature is a part of us. Scientifically, spiritually, there is this deep connection between our lives and the plants all around us.

How are you engaged with plants in your daily life? Living a vegan lifestyle, everything that I take into my body comes from this power of nature. From the whole foods encapsulated in my vegan capsules, to the foods that I eat, to the yard that gives my dogs' sanctuary, and the renewal I get every time I drive through the roads here in the Pacific Northwest. Although I felt that same renewal looking at the mountains in Utah, and enjoying the marine layers with more tropical plants on vacation. Plants give us more than we consider. And they can grow where you least expect it. My father-in-law had ivy grow through a crack in his house, into his front room. In Australia in an area where you would think nothing could grow, juniper, heather, pine, birch and (like-en) lichen still do. In areas where nothing will grow, fungi, lichen and algae partner together and create their own habitat to survive.

Essential oil use has been around, and flourishing for thousands of year, and in modern times we are just beginning to grasp the opportunities. A study done in 2003 titled IMPROVED PERFORMANCE ON CLERICAL TASKS ASSOCIATED WITH ADMINISTRATION OF PEPPERMINT ODOR. PERCEPTUAL AND MOTOR SKILLS … For well over a decade we have known that aromatherapy is the ultimate in designed biophilia. Biophilic design is connect our inherent need to affiliate with nature in the modern built environment. One of my aromatherapy instructors told us about a spa here in the Northwest that had him design a special aroma that they could use throughout the spa to take people's emotions into the forest.

No matter if you are getting into nature for a hike, playing with your dog, or simply by having a view of greenery out the window or on your desk at work there are so many applications that can be used to incorporate a biophilic design that can transform a mundane settings into stimulating environments .Applications of biophilic design are listed here. You can find more detailed descriptions in Kellert and Calabrese, The Practice of Biophilic Design (www.biophilic-design.com).

DIRECT EXPERIENCE OF NATURE

- Light
- Air
- Water
- Plants
- Animals
- Natural Landscapes and Ecosystems
- Weather

INDIRECT EXPERIENCE OF NATURE

- Images of Nature
- Natural Materials
- Natural Colors
- Mobility and Wayfinding
- Cultural and Ecological Attachment to Place
- Simulating Natural Light and Air
- Naturalistic Shapes and Forms
- Evoking Nature
- Information Richness
- Age, Change, and the Patina of Time
- Natural Geometries
- Biomimicry

As for essential oils, olfactory stimuli may be incorporated into design in several ways to support a biophilic experience.

Odorous building materials such as cedarwood can be used to integrate olfactory stimuli directly into the exposed structure and finishes of your space, contributing to its ambient scent. Mechanical systems can be programmed to appropriately administer biophilic odors via airflow to specific areas at specific times.

Vegetated areas such as herb gardens, flower boxes, water features like the urban gardens that I helped get into our school program, even just plant-lined walkways enhance spaces by designing around the source of the odor and providing access to physical interactions with nature. Design should consider the use of odor as one of many strategies to be integrated into the ecological, utilitarian, and experiential context of a space.

A multi-sensory experience amplifies the benefits of a scent and connects it with other patterns of biophilic design. The olfactory experience may be enhanced by Visual Connection with Nature, which gives context to odor; Thermal & Airflow Variability, which distributes odor throughout space; and Presence of Water and Material Connection with Nature, which each contribute to ambient odor. Olfactory stimuli may also contribute to Non-Rhythmic Sensory Stimuli with stochastic exposure to natural scents and to Mystery, which has conventionally been reserved for the visual experience, by attracting individuals using far-reaching scents. The interplay of multiple senses is essential in designing for people with limited vision or mobility, an idea realized by the Universal Design movement.

In the South Bronx, which is considered an urban desert, Stephen Ritz replaced the dirty street in front of the school with plants. He planted in desolate, empty lots throughout the community, and he brought plants into the school in order to create this connection. His non-profit, Green Bronx Machine, has evolved into K-12+ model fully integrated into core curriculum. Their students grow, eat and love their vegetables en route to spectacular academic performance. 60,000 pounds of Bronx vegetables later, he says their favorite crops include healthy students, high performing schools, graduates, registered voters, living wage jobs and members of the middle class. This is biophilia at its best.

As an aroma enthusiast, your design should consider the use of aroma as one of many strategies to be integrated into the ecological, utilitarian, and experiential context of a space. A multi-sensory experience amplifies the benefits of a scent and connects it with other patterns of biophilic design. Our olfactory experience can be enhanced by visual connection like a rosemary plant, airflow variability, like a diffuser that distributes the aroma throughout space; and I love adding that the diffuser also gives us the presence of water for our material connection with nature. Olfactory stimuli may perceptual and integrated interplay of multiple senses, and could be essential in designing for people with limited vision or mobility, an idea realized by the Universal Design movement.

For many people, you find yourself fighting to stay awake mid-afternoon with those lunch carbs safely tucked away in your belly. Diffusing the right scents in a meeting room can create a more stimulating environment and energize employees and students. A 2005 study by Phillip Zoladz and Bryan Raudenbush at Wheeling Jesuit University found that both cinnamon and peppermint scents improved participants' scores on tasks related to attentional processes, virtual recognition memory, working memory and visual-motor response speed. But study participants rated their mood and level of vigor higher and their level of fatigue lower when exposed to peppermint in particular.

Placing a few drops of Peppermint oil in a diffuser off to the side of the meeting table, or even just bringing in some sliced citrus to add to water all around the table can help re-energize us for the rest of the day. I love rubbing a drop of peppermint mixed with a carrier oil on the back of my neck, and then quickly washing my hands. Peppermint in the eye, that's no fun.

Frankincense is another one I have found that helps perk me up. Frankincense supports focused attention and tranquility. Aromatherapy for meetings should be tailored to the objectives of the gathering. Studies have found that rosemary can help improve the speed and accuracy of thinking, potentially stimulating participants learning levels.

Lavender wouldn't be the best choice for a meeting. Seventy patients were randomly assigned to a lavender oil group, a tea tree oil group, and a control group with no oil. A patient identification form, the State-Trait Anxiety Inventory, and the Pittsburgh Quality Sleep Index (PSQI) were used to measure anxiety and sleep quality before and after chemotherapy. The findings were that state anxiety before and after chemotherapy did not vary among groups. However the clinicians after comparing trait anxiety values before and after chemotherapy, they found a significant difference in the lavender group. In addition, a significant change in PSQI measurements before and after chemotherapy was observed. So knowing what your objective is for a space will help you define how you connect this bond of nature and being together.

Ever heard of Ayurvedic aromatherapy? The term "Ayurvedic Aromatherapy" has two primary meanings, being that the therapies contain aromatic plants, and therefore have essential oils as their primary active ingredients. The second is all the ways is to classify and use essential oils according to Ayurveda concepts such as Prana (life force), (oh-jas) Ojas (nutritional immunological essence), Soma (regenerative fluids), Pancha (ma-hah-bunchas) Mahabhutas (five universal elements), etc. Using this at the Chopra Center they use aromatherapy smells to relieve pain, ease anxiety, and more. All of this to me is using biophilia to reconnect us to the bond we have with nature.

The typical child in the US will now spend 90% of their time indoors. Children aged 2–5 engage in electronic media for an average of more than 30 hours per week; for 8–18-year-olds the figure is 52 hours. Most children devote just 30 minutes daily to unstructured outdoor play; a generation ago, it was more than 4 hours. Many parents fear letting their children play outdoors on their own, and see learning as a formal indoor process. The body of evidence that has been gathered from US, European and Australian studies showcases that this disconnection may be causing physical, emotional and intellectual deficits in our children's learning and development.

A young child engaged in free play in a grove of trees or under a garden bush experiences a wealth of kinetic, aural, visual and tactile stimulation. These experiences foster a wide array of adaptive responses that provoke curiosity, observation, wonder, exploration, problem-solving and creativity. A child building a dam or den gains understanding of gradients, forces, materials, the behavior of water and wood, and the local environment. The centrality of nature in children's learning begins with our origins as a species. For more than 99% of our evolutionary history, humans adapted in response to mainly natural forces.

A study of 90 schools for children aged 5 to 12 in Australia, for example, found that being outdoors improved the children's self-confidence, ability to work with others, caring, peer relationships and interaction with adults (C. Maller and M. Townsend Int. J. Learn. 12, 359–372; 2006).The natural world is more than a decorative backdrop or a dispensable amenity. Experiencing it is an act of profound self-interest, a guard against a future as imperiling to the long-term fitness of our species as the more obvious threats of poverty and disease. Alan Ewert's classic 1989 book Outdoor Adventure Pursuits (Gorsuch Scarisbrick) reviewed studies of children participating in nature programs, and found that these children asked more questions than others, and were better at solving problems.

A study of 262 children aged 3–12 in poor neighborhoods in Chicago, Illinois, demonstrated richer creative play following exposure to nature (A. Faber Taylor et al. Environ. Behav. 30, 3–27; 1998).Nature is an essential part of what we need in our lives, and what changes the pathways of our brain in the essential development stages. In the UK pediatric experts found that Aromatherapy was effective for promoting infant healing and neonatal abstinence syndrome (NAS) recovery in the neonatal intensive care unit using Lavender essential oil on a floppy green pillow. Babies receive aromatherapy as part of their medical treatment, Daniel applied thumbnail-size patch to the "palm" of a floppy green pillow called a Zaky arm. The Zaky arms, which mimic the feeling and shape of a caregiver's arm, carry both the scent of the baby's mother and calming aromatherapy oils. He then placed the Lavender-scented pillow alongside a baby dozing off in a NICU bed.

Herbalists, chemists and massage therapists have long professed the therapeutic and healing properties of essential oils. Lavender oil, which produces the mood-balancing serotonin chemical in the brain, triggers sedative states and relaxation while chamomile oil balances out emotions. Dr. Lori Shook and Dr. John Daniel completed a pilot study reporting positive results from administering aromatherapy as an adjunctive treatment for babies recovering from NAS. These preliminary results showed that babies who received aromatherapy stayed in the NICU an average of 6.4 fewer days than babies who did not receive the aromatherapy treatment. The doctors found babies who received aromatherapy also needed smaller doses of withdrawal maintenance medication than those who didn't receive aromatherapy.

Shortening an NAS infant's length of stay in the NICU helps families, but also reduces medical costs. One day of treatment in the NICU nursery costs about $5,000 for one baby. The study suggests that aromatherapy patches, at about two dollars apiece, can be implemented cost-effect measure for reducing drawn-out hospital admission for NAS treatment. Nature and development is part of what makes this such vital information to pass along.

The most important thing you can take away from this book is that what is around us matters so much more than we realize. The EMF from the cells phones stuck to our heads all day long, which may keep us connected to our family and friends, however they are taking collateral damages along the way. The fact that we see more trees being cut down to create formaldehyde homes will come back to haunt us in the future. As well, beyond that, the synthetic aromas and food products that we are devouring as a nation are not truly raising our serotonin levels in our brains. Rather these lab created items are destroying our gut, and that in turn is lowering our natural serotonin levels. Sugar is not happiness, faux lemon oil neither. What you connect to, as a body, is meant to be in alignment with this Earth. Being in nature is aligned to our entire being just because we, too, are nature.

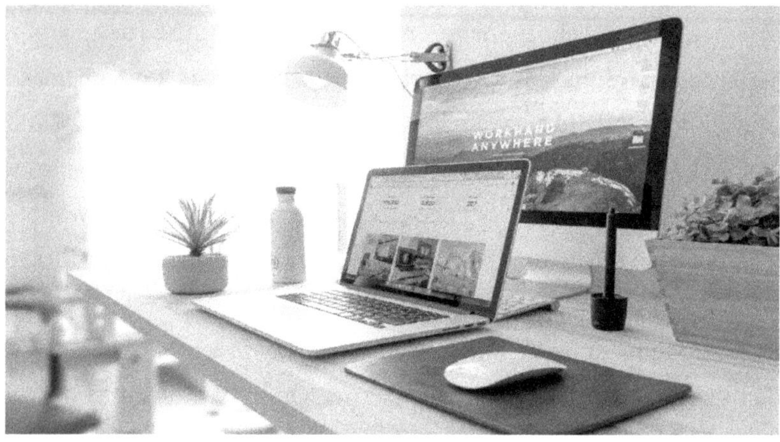

Don't just look at nature on your screen. Be in nature as often as you can. And when you cannot be in nature, bring nature in and create a natural zone.

7

METHODS OF USE

What are the different ways in which you can use essential oils and why?

"Risk needs to be balanced with benefit. If every substance that has caused at least on allergic reaction was forbidden in personal care products, there would be no personal care products, and if every essential oil was used at a level that presented zero risk, there might be no benefits at all."
Robert Tisserand

Essential oil use has been around, and flourishing for thousands of year, and in modern times we are just beginning to grasp the possibility of what is possible. While safety should always factor into use with essential oils, it is important to understand that there are many ways of using oils, and that no one way is the right way for all. Although there are a lot of opinions on which oil is the best, and a lot of opinions on buying oils from network marketing companies, my opinion is that a company that tests and shares those results with transparency, goes out into the globe to verify safe practices, and that has a lot to lose by selling poor quality oils… that's the company to buy from.

When starting an aroma practice it is important to balance holistic ethics with your desires. Do no harm is the most important and first tenet we practice when sharing aroma with others. That means exploring what is truly needed from the aroma, and what the best method of use is for the person using the oil or oil blend. This also means you must be mindful of yourself and the reaction you are noticing as you are selecting or recommending an essential oil for use.

Be Professional. This means you must present yourself with integrity and honesty, as well as a respect for others.

Know your scope of practice. There isn't a government program of adherence for those using essential oils beyond they do not treat, cure, prevent or provide use as a drug or in a medical nature. Consider this as you work with others to share your excitement for essential oils.

When using essential oils for aromatherapy for any part of your practice, you must have consent to do so. As a therapeutic addition to any other modality, make sure you get permission and guidelines from your client as to how they want the essential oils use. This informed consent can be either oral or in writing and should provide accurate information to the client regarding the nature of your use of essential oils.

Clients expect that you will keep their confidentiality and all manners related to your work with them. It can be especially complex for those with dual relationships as both social friends, and professional relationships. Create that agreement for both confidentiality and a boundary that separates and defines these different relationships.

As many energy workers are very empathic, set up a boundary for yourself that you will not allow transference of energy, unconscious or not, from thoughts, feelings and beliefs from your client to your own being. This includes from their life, past or present.

Use of carrier oils is important with most methods of essential oil use. What the term carrier oil means is any oil that you may use to help dilute your essential oil and to help move the oil through the skin layers upon application. Selecting a cold-pressed carrier or expeller-pressed oil gives you an oil that retains its most valuable properties. Anytime oil is refined it changes its composition. Unrefined oils are minimally processed using pressure and lower temperatures. You may hear these called virgin or extra-virgin in the marketplace. Choosing a carrier oil can be as complex as selecting the essential oil itself.

The oils you will see used the most for at home aromatherapy will be the same oils you may use for cooking. Coconut oil, olive oil, avocado oil and sesame oil are often the oils you will use. Perhaps you may use some aloe leaves to provide you with a carrier product, or for your skin you may use jojoba or grapeseed oil. An important note for aloe vera is that it is not recommended for use with anyone that has a natural latex sensitivity due to its natural latex properties. Carrier oil quality and how a client will react to a carrier oil matters just as much as the quality of your essential oil. Consider the shelf life of your carrier oil and any allergies of your client before creating an oil blend. Diluting your essential oil, as well, is a mandatory part of the essential oil practice, and learning about the carrier oils can enhance both safety and help you create extra benefits to your end product.

It is essential to do a skin patch test before using any essential oil in any manner that will come in contact with the body, outside of aromatherapy diffusion. Most of us will never experience any type of adverse reaction, yet some will. Having a reaction to an essential oil can have simple or serious consequences. Reactions to essential oils can include irritation, allergic hypersensitivity, and contact urticaria (pronounced er-ticka-ria) which is an immediate but transient localized swelling and redness that occurs on the skin after direct contact with an offending substance. Urticaria is often a wheal or flare reaction and/or eczema following external contact with a substance, usually appearing within 30 minutes and clearing completely within hours, typically without residual signs. That is why it is important to watch the area, and not just slap a Band-Aid on and call it good. As well it is best to go with a latex-free bandage as essential oils degrade latex, and degrading a substance that can be absorbed into the skin and cause a later hypersensitivity is not the result you want with skin testing.

This reaction usually happens with most people within five to ten minutes. They may say they feel burning or pain, show tiny hives developing, or just redness and/or itching. To wash off an irritating essential oil apply more of the carrier oil to a cotton ball, tissue, or handkerchief and gently wipe to dilute and remove the oil from the skin. Make sure you use a carrier oil that would not be the allergic offender. People often find reactions due to undiluted or insufficiently diluted essential oils placed on the skin.

This also often happens when undiluted or poorly diluted essential oils are added to a bath. Sometimes a reaction may happen in the form of delayed hypersensitivity, like we see with latex allergies. Considered a Type 4 hypersensitivity the reaction takes several days to develop, or develops after repeated exposure. This type of reaction is not antibody-mediated but rather is a type of cell-mediated response. Once the essential oil has penetrated the skin, it binds to peptides at the surface of the Langerhans cells. These cells then migrate to the local lymph nodes where cytotoxic T lymphocytes stand primed for immune defense. These cells travel to the epidermis where these CD8+ T cells are recruited to the allergen-exposed site and initiate the inflammatory process leading to skin infiltration with subsequent applications. If you have atopic dermatitis you are at a greater risk of this sort of oil irritation. Also those with seasonal allergies or that are prone to skin allergens may already have had these immune-reaction cells migrate throughout the body causing an allergic reaction.

For those that apply and use a lot of essential oils, especially orally and topically, this can cause a reaction due to the overuse of the oils and the way you use them. Memory CD8+ T Cells are an essential component of our long-term immunity because of their longevity and their special ability to rapidly expand in numbers to go after the offender on secondary antigen encounters. Think of it in terms of those that are gluten sensitive due to memory B cells being created from eating wheat. There are studies taking place to see if essential oils can be used as Immunomodulators. This is why it is important to understand essential oil safety, and to test, especially essential for children, those with compromised immune systems and the elderly. Still important for us all to always be cautious.

The skin patch test and contraindications of specific essential oils are indicated before all essential oil use beyond aroma diffuser.

HOW TO DO A SKIN PATCH TEST

Use a 0.25-0.5 dilution for your skin patch testing. Mix 1-2 drops of the appropriate essential oil to 4 tsp of carrier oil. Apply a drop of this mixture one inch below the inner elbow and cover with a latex-free bandage. Wait and watch for 24 hours. Essential oils degrade latex over time.

USING ESSENTIAL OILS SAFELY

Using oils in baths is a simple, effective and gentle way to relax and receive the therapeutic benefits of essential oils. Water itself has therapeutic value, which enhances the powers of the oils. Adding one to just a few drops of the right essential oil with the right emulsifier can enhance the bathing experience. The effects of a full-body bath will vary according to the temperature of the water and the duration of time the individual will be in the water. Your essential oils or hydrosols should be added to the bath once you are in it, and not added while the water is running. Once the individual is in the bath, add the appropriate essential oil drops that have been combined with a dispersant. The body picks up a very thin, even layer of oil as you enter a bath and it guards against a whole drop of oil settling on the skin, which can be slightly irritating. When essential oils are put directly into bath water without a dispersing agent, they can harm the skin because essential oils are soluble with the lipid membranes of cells.

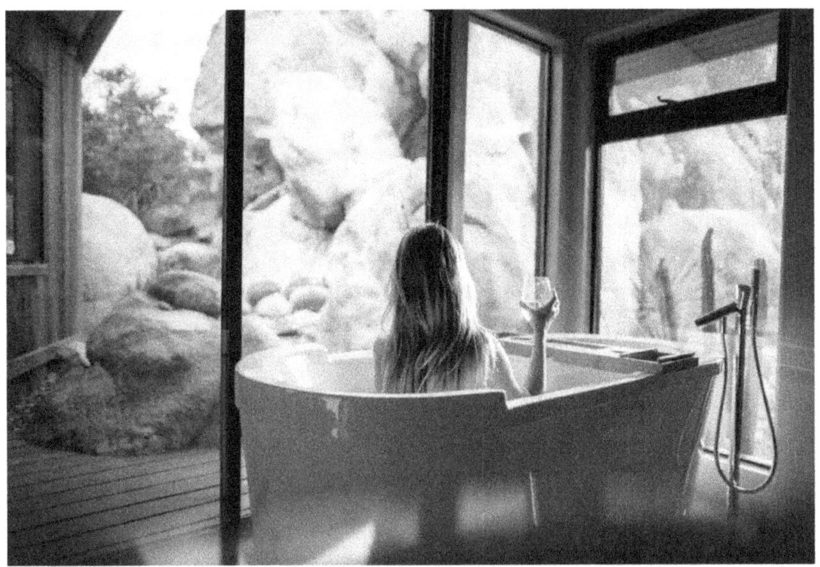

Never add your undiluted essential oils directly to bath water. For aromatherapy add only 1 and up to 4 drops of essential oils in 2 tablespoons of carrier so that the oils spread evenly over the surface. Placing essential oils in the bath prior to immersion can lose some of the desired effects, as well as increase the chance of irritation to the mucous membranes of the vaginal and/or rectal area. Avoid essential oils that are dermal irritants, dermal sensitizers, and mucus membrane irritants in baths

Similarly to how nicotine and hormone skin patches rely on transdermal absorption to deliver drugs into the bloodstream, essential oils have an ability to disperse within minutes throughout the body when absorbed through the skin.

Since oil and water don't mix, this application of essential oils can be very challenging. The most beneficial way to use a drop to four drops of the essential oil is to add your diluted product to a cup of

Epsom salts. This allows the oil to disperse more evenly, and prevents some of the stronger oils from being irritating to sensitive areas.

General bath time for a full-body hot bath at 100 degrees F is 20 minutes or less. Using the Epson salt bath with those that have high blood pressure or a salt sensitivity is to be avoided.

Alternating hot and cold sitz baths are often recommended for those that desire relieving congestion in the female reproductive area, helping with hemorrhoids or to ease constipation. You find this more with European nature cure practitioners using a pump, but for this practice we are talking about have two bowls large enough to sit in. One would be filled with hot water and one with cold. You may add a drop with carrier oil to each bowl. Sit in one, and place your feet in the other, splash the water over your abdomen. After 30 seconds to a minute, change position and repeat.

When using essential oils in a plastic fiberglass tub some essential oils can cause staining. A full-body bath is defined as —the complete immersion of the body in a fluid or in a vaporous medium such as steam‖ (Green 2000, p. 254).

There are four simple guidelines to choosing a warm compress or a cold compress.

- Use Cold Therapy immediately after an injury to reduce inflammation.
- Do not use Cold Therapy on stiff muscles or joints.
- Use Hot Therapy to relax/soothe sore muscles or to increase range of motion.

- Do not use Hot Therapy on an injury that is already warm to the touch.

A compress can be as simple as cotton or flannel cloth that has been soaked in cold/hot water. Soak and then wring out the excess water and apply directly to the affected part. Compresses are usually for the help with small localized areas. I often use a warm washcloth compress on my sinus areas in the morning and to help dry eyes get going. Cold aromatic compresses can be applied with the standard sports related RICE. RICE stands for: REST, ICE, COMPRESS, ELEVATE. This is a sports related technique for the relief of recent sprains, strains, and bruising, swelling and inflammation, sprains with swelling but can also be used with bug bites. I often make a paste out of a drop of essential oil and baking soda to place on a bug bite. You can make a cold compress using cold water with ice added. Once it is wrapped in wrap, add an ice pack.

Hot compress as usually used in cases of pain relief for such conditions as menstrual cramps, muscle aches and pains or bruises. You could also use it for eczema or psoriasis. I recently had a latex-related allergic reaction that caused a skin eczema flare up. I found that a cold compress was best for me, so use what feels right for your body. For a warm compress fill a large glass jar with as hot a water as you or your child can stand, add the drops of essential oils, put the lid on jar and shake well to disperse the oil. Pour the hot water into a large bowl and soak a cotton cloth or cloth diaper in the water, wring out and lay over the area. Wrap up, and you can add a warm towel as it will help to keep your compress warm. When cool, redo the compress following same procedure. A hot compress can also increase blood flow to a particular part of the body.

Cold Packs: Apply 1 – 2 drops of essential oils in a little bit of carrier, followed by cold water or ice packs when helping with inflamed or swollen tissues. Frozen packages of peas or corn make excellent ice packs that will mold to the contours of the body part and will not leak. Keep the cold pack on until the swelling diminishes. For neurological support, always use cold packs, never hot.

HOT PACKS: Apply 1 – 2 drops of essential oils in a little bit of carrier. For deeper penetration of an essential oil, use hot packs. Start by dipping a cloth in comfortably hot water. Wring the cloth out and place it on location. After allowing it to cool, wrap it loosely with another dry towel or blanket to seal in the heat. Use this technique 1 – 3 times daily as needed.

ADDING ESSENTIAL OILS TO YOUR SKIN CARE ROUTINE

Essential oils can't get rid of wrinkles, but they can help minimize them. Essential oils are very concentrated. Dilute all essential oils before applying to the skin, either in a fatty oil or in water as when used on a compress.

Since becoming a Certified Aromatherapist I have seen a lot of essential oils transitioning to everyday products like skin care. Essential oils can rejuvenate the skin and promote smoother complexion, however used improperly can cause damage. The trick is finding which ones work for you, because like any skin product, different types of essential oils have different functional abilities.

When adding essential oils to your facial or body cleanser choose the correct essential oils for your skin type and blend them in with an ordinary unperfumed brand of cleanser, liquid soap, or tissue-off lotion/cream. For 25 mls. of product you can use base notes – 1 drop per 25 mls., middle notes 3 drops per 25 mls. , top notes 4 drops per 25 mls. You can also find beautifully simplistic bars of soap that use essential oils in them. My bath bar is a hemp based bar with tea tree essential oil added. Adding a drop of oil to water after your skin has been cleansed with a konjac sponge, or in the toner is another option.

When adding an oil into a facial oil or facial serum, use carrier oils rich in (lin-oh-lee-ic) linoleic acid, for example pericarp oil, grapeseed oil, rosehip oil or evening primrose oil. I love using Pericarp oil because the mangosteen seed contains essential vitamins for our bodies, including linoleic acid (LA) and alpha-linoleic acid (LNA) - with linoleic acid being the most complete fatty acid. There are two basic categories of EFA's (essential fatty acids) - omega-3 and omega-6 which include linoleic acid and gamma-linoleic acid. Omega fatty acids truly are remarkable ingredients for skin. They serve as the essential building blocks of skin's surface layers, creating a smoother, more even, younger-looking, and healthier complexion, no matter your age or skin type.

Essential oils are the gentlest way of toning your skin. Rose water for normal or dry/sensitive skin or witch hazel for oilier skin is an ideal base for fresheners. These can be applied with cotton wool or for a more refreshing tone, sprayed on to the face. Herbal tea infusions can also be used as toners. Boil a cup of water and infuse chamomile, marigold or even rosehip herbs or herbal tea bags to make it simple. Do not use chamomile or marigold with people who have ragweed allergies. Add your tea to a glass bottle. Oils you can add include Orange or Lavender essential oil. Orange essential oil: 20 drops to 100 mls.of infusion. Lavender essential oil: 15 drops to 100 mls.of infusion. Oily skins benefit from Juniper whereas drier skins would appreciate Rose or Sandalwood. Allow your infusion to cool before using.

An aromatherapy foot massage is a great way to help a child or an adult unwind after an active day and prepare them for sleep. It is also a good home remedy for aching muscles when you have been overactive or to aid your child while participating in school sports programs when diluted properly.

Any aromatherapy application can release toxins or hormones from the tissues, especially the tissues of the arms, legs and buttocks – areas which have given shelter to unwanted body wastes and other poisons. As they are released, they must be eliminated from the body via the lymphatic system, blood stream, kidneys, bladder and digestive systems. The process of elimination will cause spots and blemishes to appear on the surface of the skin where aromatherapy application is being given. This is different from a non-diluted rash. Whichever route is used in the elimination process, it must be encouraged to flow at a steady pace. If too many toxins are released into the body's circulation at the same time, too great a strain can be put on the organs of elimination. This can result in toxins either being reabsorbed into the body again, or being unable to be eliminated quickly, circulating in the bloodstream and possibly resulting in some of what has been called "detox symptoms". Refer back to your skin test to make sure that you are not dealing with an oil that is not a topical fit for your body.

Steam inhalation is generally thought of as being used specifically for the respiratory system but can be effectively applied to support the expectorating properties of essential oils. Steam encourages better product absorption and releases toxins. It is important to note that the person will be inhaling the steam into their lungs and nose and mouth. Boyd and Sheppard (1968) report that steam inhalation can affect the output and composition of respiratory tract fluid. They also point out that low dilutions of aromatics for short periods of time are most effective. This method is great for head colds and sinus ailments. My ND recommends a drop added to a large mug of warm water in order to support healthy respiratory functions. Longer exposure times can reduce the efficacy of steam inhalations so short durations and low concentrations are the keys to optimal results.

For skin care use a 1 or 2 oz. bottle or vial, few grains of Icelandic rock salt (Do not use for people who have high blood pressure) to help disperse the essential oil well. Bring 2 cups of water to boil, reduce heat, and let water cool just a bit for 5 to 10 minutes. Pour water into a glass bowl and place on a table so the individual can sit or stand with a towel over their head, over the bowl and inhale the steam. Please remember not to get your face too close to the hot steam and please be careful not to knock over your bowl. Add 1 to 4 drops of essential oil and stir to disperse evenly. Inhale vapors for 3 to 5 minutes. A towel can be placed over the head to increase the concentration of inhalation. Inhalations can be used 2 or 3 times a day when supporting specific respiratory wellness. Essential oils can help maintains a feeling of a clear airway and easy breathing while minimizing the effects of seasonal threats. You can use you could use Rosemary, Eucalyptus Radiata, or Peppermint depending on contraindications of these essential oils. Always be aware of these issues we discussed earlier in this program. Chamomile if you don't have ragweed allergies is a wonderful essential oil. Chamomile is a powerhouse of antioxidants and protects the skin from free-radical damage. Lavender, Peppermint and Rosemary can be stimulating. Parsley, Geranium and Fennel are all also very wonderful for skin support. As I licensed cosmetologist I regularly steamed my face starting in my early 20's and believe that is part of my secret to younger looking skin.

THERAPEUTIC DILUTION RECOMMENDATIONS

A low concentration of 1 – 4 drops of essential oil or a blend of essential oils in total sum equals 4 drops of essential oil at the most in approximately 2 cups of steaming hot water is sufficient. The steam should feel soothing, not burning. Add three drops of the oil you select for a soothing steam in a basin of water. Place a towel over the client's head and ask him or her to inhale for ten minutes. Remember to ask the client to close his or her eyes and remove spectacles and contact lenses. Contact lenses can absorb some of the essential oil and cause stinging. It is a good idea to remove lenses before steam inhalation.

You may follow up your steam session by applying toner with a cotton ball as this will cleanse away extra dirt that has been loosened from your pores. Apply your regular moisturizer to lock in moisture and protect your skin from the sun if leaving outdoors afterwards, or if you have used photosensitive oils. If photosensitive oil is applied to the skin and then you expose it to sunlight or UV rays you risk the chances of skin discoloration in mild cases to burning and blistering in more severe cases. Using photosensitive oils at nighttime helps reduce the risks associated with these oils.

CAUTION: Keep eyes closed to avoid irritation. Avoid mucus membrane irritating essential oils. Check throughout the program to see which ones are mucus membrane irritating. Avoid this procedure with the elderly, confused, very young, or infirm.

When you want to clean out those pores both clay and certified gluten-free oatmeal is an ideal ingredient for any face mask and whole body clay pack. Natural powdered calcium bentonite clay is also an amazing choice. This can be mixed into a paste with hot water. Once cool you can add plain yogurt for a smoother consistency. Similarly, finely ground oatmeal can be mixed into a paste and left to cool. Add drops of essential oils to suit your skin type per cupful of paste. Smooth on to your face, leave to dry slightly and then sponge off. For particularly dry/sensitive skins add one tablespoon of evening primrose base oil to give a more moisturizing mask. When applying, avoid the eye area. Always make sure you gently remove the mask with an organic muslin cloth. Gently swab the skin after with a cotton wool soaked in your floral water toner and apply a little facial oil to return some oils back into your skin.

Facial masks should not be used too often as they will draw out not only impurities from the skin, but also the skin's natural oils. Exfoliation too often will cause dry skin to become even drier. There are very few natural skin care exfoliation products that are actually healthy for you skin. I generally use a very protective gel that gently renews my skin without any grains, abrasives, or acids. Other more abrasive masks should be used once a month.

Oils are often promoted for dehydrated dry skin, because of the lack of natural oils. That means that dry skin requires daily feeding with protective and nourishing oils. Without these the skin will becomes wrinkled more easily. Select oils for their ability to improve the condition of dry skin and remember to apply to both the face and neck. Dryness of the skin can also be caused by living in our modern centrally-heated homes, through your office building, overuse of sun tanning; an imbalance of vitamins and minerals, also due to hormonal changes during the menopause or pregnancy. Even added stress, pollutants and of course; smoking can cause drier skin tones. Oils that are wonderful for drier skin include Geranium, Rose and New Caledonia Sandalwood. If you are more sensitive to topically applied oils, I recommend trying German Chamomile, True Lavender or a blend of Ylang Ylang complete, Bergamot, Cypress, Rosemary, and Helichrysum can help moisturize severely-dry skin. Frankincense can rejuvenate and hydrate your skin as well. As a licensed cosmetologist I know that dry skin is becoming more and more prevalent.

Nothing could be more perfect than aromatherapy for helping with acneic complexions. My first experience with this was using tea tree as a young adult. Essential oils that have wonderful ability to pass through the skin barrier via the fluids and penetrate into the body. Many essential oils are cleansing and antibacterial. Juniper berry, Tea Tree and Clary Sage are a few of my favorite oils that you may find in many of your organic acne products. Even Good Housekeeping and Reader's Digest have been recommending essential oils as natural alternatives for acne flare ups. As a reminder, most acne is caused by clogged pores. Excess oil production, bacteria, and excess hormonal activity are causes as well. Since diet can be a factor, it's always important to look at what else could be the cause. Even stress can be an acne trigger. I prefer to use Frankincense on my skin a lot of time. Not only is it a wonderful healing resin, but is also a very soothing oil to help dismiss feelings of nervousness or tension. It is a wonderful way to start the day, or wind down in the evening.

Combination Skin is the skin that has that oily T-zone panel from the forehead down to the nose and chin area, and may be normal or dry elsewhere. Oil blends are best for these areas.

Finally at the end of the day, sometimes all you need is a nice cool eye compress. Tired eyes, or those irritated by contact lenses or a smoky atmosphere, will find immediate relief from a Chamomile or Lavender essential oil or rose water eye compress. Never do spicy oils or oils like Peppermint near your eyes. It's lovely to do an eye compress in conjunction with a face mask.

Add one drop of essential oil into a 500 ml. bottle of spring water and shake well. After soaking two cotton wool pads in the liquid, squeeze out excess water and place a pad over each eye. Maybe even place a few slices of cucumber on your eyes like at the spa if you are looking for something special for those tired eyes. The flesh of cucumbers contains vitamin C and caffeic acid, which both help soothe skin irritations and reduce swelling.

Essential oils can often bring things to the surface, as can hormones and many other things in life. Crying can be beneficial and can release a lot of stored emotions and energy. Think of it like spring cleaning your house. Puffy red eyes can be soothed and made to regain their normal appearance quickly by applying a Lavender or Chamomile essential oil compress to each eye. Do not use Chamomile if you are allergic to ragweed. Use a piece of cotton wool about the size of the palm of your hand (so that the compress is large enough not only to cover the immediate eye area but also to help with any puffiness to the upper cheeks and the area up to and including the eyebrows). If possible, lie down for half an hour with some Reiki or frequency music from YouTube playing in the background. Add one drop of essential oil into a 500 ml. bottle of spring water and shake well. After soaking two cotton wool pads in the liquid, squeeze out excess water and place a pad over each eye. Use same recipe as above for eye compresses. Always remove contact lenses before using your eye compress.

You can make your own rose water at home with ease. It takes a whopping 10,000 pounds of rose petals to make a single pound of rose essential oil. Rose tea is made from entire rose buds, so it contains the nutrients found in the rose hips as well as the petals. Use a handful of fresh rose tea free of pesticide residue, or similar organic rose tea into a pot. Add just enough distilled water to cover them. Don't use tap water because the ph has the potential to change the color and aroma of the roses. Cover the pot and bring the contents to a boil, being quick to reduce temperature to a simmer for 20 to 30 minutes. Strain the mixture (cheesecloth or nut bag, but a fine metal mesh strainer works) to remove the petals. Pour the rose water into a glass jar. Seal the jar. Once it cools to room temperature, refrigerate it where it can be used for a month or for a week if you store it at room temperature.

What you see on your hands (and everywhere else on your body) are really dead skin cells or the epidermis. The outer layer and the dermis inner layer are the largest organ of the body. How you care for it, and what you put on it is very important. Skin is that secondary chimney passageway to remove toxins from the body and helps prevent chemical and waste build-up in support of your primary chimney. Part of the reason we have skin oils is to fight off disease. The subtle body flows inside our skin, tissues and glands, and several of our auras emanate from our skin outwards.

In the practice of Subtle Aromatherapy you combine two forms of healing—aromatherapy, and subtle energy therapy. Essential oils can affect all layers of our energy body-physical, emotional, mental and spiritual. They can protect the outer edges of the field by forming a protective shield around us and so it is only natural to consider the benefits of topical oil applications.

Possibly the most popular way of using inhalation in a health-care setting at the moment is from a diffuser. This method can be used to purify the air when infectious illness is around. It can also be used to rid the air of cooking smells, subtly influence mood – or simply create a delightful ambience in the home or workplace. This must be one of the most enjoyable applications of essential oils, and involves vaporizing the oils in a variety of devices into the air that we breathe. This differs from having synthetically fragranced potpourri placed around a room. Since with essential oil vaporization, you get both the benefit of a fragrant smelling room, plus the benefits of the therapeutic effects of the essential oils.

Diffusion refers to the method of transmitting essential oils into the air within a specified area. One of the simplest ways to quickly diffuse the scent of essential oils is to place a few drops on a tissue and place it near the space you are occupying such as a desk, chair or bed. The scent will not be overpowering and will last a short time. You can replenish the oil on the tissue as needed. Vapor therapy is a simple technique using droplets of essential oil on a tissue or handkerchief and smelling it at intervals for the desired effect.

Diffusers are used to project the scent into a room in a fast and efficient way. Diffusing therapeutic oils into a room has been done for centuries. Diffused oils alter the structure of molecules that create odors, rather than just masking them. They also produce negative ions. Many essential oils, such as lemon can cleanse and purify the air and surfaces in the home. Lemon also contains a clean, fragrant scent that makes it perfect for diffusing. Diffusers put the essential oils into the atmosphere and start healing almost instantly. Place the diffuser in a dry and cool place.

Regular ultrasonic diffusers allow you to place a drop or two of oils into a container of water, and when turned on send evaporated water particles out to transport the essential oil into the room. A nebulizer processes your essential oils into an almost gas like state. The oil bottle is generally attached directly to the nebulizing diffuser. This releases the small oil particles into the air so that they are more easily absorbed by your body.

Diffusing is a natural, non-toxic way to calm your nerves and help you to relax without the side effects of medications and drugs. The aroma penetrates your bloodstream and into your central control system to alter brain functions and your mood. Hence, you can reduce anxiety in an instant and improving other brain functions such as concentration and focus. This method has been used quite successfully in a group aromatherapy sessions, in classrooms and afternoon meetings.

There are also aromatherapy oil burners that vaporize essential oil and they are becoming more popular. These oil burners provide a relaxed and soothing atmosphere at home or a supportive environment for mental sharpness and creativity in an office setting.

I also place a few drops of essential oil on a small ball of cotton wool, and then place it in my dryer, but you could also place it in your drawers,. Just make sure in your dresser that it does not touch your clothes, since the oil may stain.

All essential oils have different properties. Oils like Bergamot, Lavender and Ylang Ylang help to relax and unwind after a stressful day while Black Pepper, Lemon and Rosemary revitalize a wary mind. When you are irritable or your energy level is low Chamomile and Lavender are essential oils that will relieve stress and calm the nerves. These oils can be used alone or combined for a potent mix to relieve irritability. You will be refreshed and energized after just a few days of using these essential oils in your diffuser, and they can be purchased for very little. Diffusing essential oils promotes relaxation, relieves tension, clears the mind and improves concentration, alertness and mental clarity and can improve your concentration in your office or help your children focus on their homework after school. Always diffuse in a well-ventilated area and make sure that what you're diffusing is safe for pets, children, or anyone else who may be around.

Refer to Chapter One for a refresher on Top, Middle and Base Notes and the typically evaporation time when using different weights of oils for aromatherapy.

7

PLANT SPIRITS

What is a spirit? It relates to nothing material, not to our soul, and not to our emotions. When we talk about a spirit it isn't just some unknown force in the atmosphere, but it is an energy that shapes everything around us, and yet isn't physically there.

What is a plant spirit? Disease within energy practices is believed to originate from an imbalance or disharmony in our emotional and spiritual energy, and that plants are effective in healing these bodies. Tribal shamans have long been considered to be the spiritual liaisons between the plants and the spirit world. Plant Spirits are the consciousness and healing properties of plants that shamanic healers connect with on an energy level.

As we have discussed, our growth, our cells, our being is very compatible with nature. Starting with our first ancestors, there have been rituals, traditions, teachings and lore that are deeply connected to the plant spirit. So what is a plant spirit? A plant spirit is nothing more than the energy of the plants that shamanic healers tune into on an energy level to liaison between the plants, the spirit world and us.

The energy of what we call spirit is everywhere, and in everything. When you become aware of the spirit of a plant, you can tune into any guidance it may give to help you in your blends and herbal preparations. This may be as simple as using smell to determine if your body desires and oil, or it can be as complex as learning to directly access your own balance and needs.

This idea is deeply connected to our relationship with the Earth, and how rooted our energy systems are with the Earth. The Earth and everything connected to it is our connection, our vital source, our physical life, our nutrients and minerals, and the very core of our survival and existence.

Mala is Sanskrit for 'root', and Adhara is Sanskrit for 'base'. The Muladhara is the name for your root chakra. There is a deeper reason that we are vitally rooted through nature, walking barefoot outdoors, visually attuned to being in nature, and feel a deeper connection to the inner knowing that this world is home.

If we slow ourselves down and allow ourselves to feel our true being outside of what we consider to be this physical plane, can you feel an ending to your being? Do you see how intertwined your energy is with everything, including these plants. Plants become like friends when we open up to this understanding, and we relax when we are around them.

How do I know that we have a relationship with plants? First off the way a plant grows can be influenced by the way we talk and nurture them, which has been proven by science. Plants pick up on our inner voices, and so they know beyond what you have said to them. Plants can sense and react to so many changes like temperature, weather, and even human touch. And a study showed that although they have no specialized structure to perceive sound like we do, plants can discern the sound of predators through tiny vibrations of their leaves, and will increase their defenses in response.

Secondly, everything around us consists of vibrational frequencies and energy. We may not be able to teleport like Scotty from Star Trek yet, but our energy can. Have you ever heard of photosynthesis? This is how plants are able to harvest as much as 95 percent of the sunlight they soak up, instantly converting solar energy into chemical energy, and it happens in 1 million billionth of a second. That plants use quantum mechanics to achieve this near-perfect efficiency is something mind blowing. They do this using the quantum principle of superposition, which is being in many different places at the same time. In an amazing study scientists found that plants absorb energy from other plants as well. The biological research team at Bielefeld University showed that plants can draw an alternative source of energy from other plants. When we talk about people and plants drawing from each other's energy it has been called Empathic blending, and it is everything that plant spirits and plant medicine are about.

When you listen to your oils, or the plants you are talking to, you must set a clear intention of being one with the spirit of the plant. Hippocrates, said, "Let food be thy medicine, and medicine thy food." It feels like that statement goes deeper than that. We are atoms that are exchanging electrons with other atoms around us, as Tesla learned. The best place to start practicing this conversation with nature is out in nature first. When you sit in a space where you feel grounded, grateful, open and ready to receive, it seems to open your chakras to a knowing. What do you feel pulled towards? Be aware of that, because that is the sense of how you will distinguish which oil you are being pulled to use.

Spend some time trying to converse with nature… I know it sounds really weird to hear someone say that out loud, but words are just vocal energy, and thoughts are measurable if you want to think and not speak. No reason to look crazy at this point. Look for its biomagnetic energy field, this is called the aura. The lower aura frequencies are connected to what we visualize as our metabolism and circulation. The higher frequencies then are what we visualize as our conscious and subconscious minds. The etheric body, or subtle body is the first or lowest layer in our aura. It is said to be in immediate contact with the physical body, to sustain it and connect it with "higher" bodies. Your first connection with other energies goes through the subtle body, and we will discuss this deeper in another section of this course. Know that a plant just like a human has an auric field.

Listen to what surrounds you, and how you feel. Just like you can empathic connect to the emotions and dreams of someone around you, the empath can feel the emotions and dream state of the plant world. If you are ready to work with the plant, perhaps to make some pine needle tea, make your intention known. See if the tree is open to you using its needles for your wellness journey. You should feel an energy of what the plant's answer is. Open heart, warmth, flowing energy is an opportunity to start working together. Feeling cold, experiencing negative emotions or anything that feels like the breaks are being put on should be understood as a no. Yes and no are like truth and lies. One feels light and the other feels heavy. As you know if you have worked in the energy realm, no isn't what we perceive as no. It means perhaps not know, what other awareness are you having, what question haven't you asked, what else is possible about what you want to accomplish?

Getting to know nature is about experiencing their world, their textures, formation, growth or retreat, in a community of others, or a lone wolf. Does it desire love, compassion, or just to be left alone for now. Does looking at the plant, touching the plant remind you of anything? Listen, smell, watch, touch, and with many herbs you can taste. Similarly with essential oils. for those into herbs and nature, you can create a book of notes and sketches to help guide you in working with other plant spirits. When you have finished working with a plant spirit, always leave with gratitude and truth. Those that work highly in plant spiritualism you can also learn to listen to the body's energy imbalance and call upon the spirit of plants to correct the imbalance.

HARMONIOUS ENERGIES

Yin and Yang are two independent yet complementary energies. They represent energies so vast that they encompass everything in the universe. Yin and Yang cannot exist without the other; they are never separate. Traditional Chinese medical philosophies and shamanic healers both work with the five elements. The Five Elements are Wood, Earth, Water, Fire, and Metal. They are seen as generating each other in a never ending cycle that never remains static. Life beings connect with Yin. Yang is contained in Yin and these two forces can only be defined in relationship to each other. Plant medicine is about bringing Yin and Yang back into balance. Yin and Yang as the five elements are actually just Qi, or life force. Life force energy animates our physical form. The Earth Element is the densest of the five elemental energies. Earth elements allow us to open up to the natural spiritual wisdom that abounds around us.

The five elements are also used in energy work to and are called the five (/'tʌtvə/) Tattwa symbols. Tattwa are geometric images from India. They are symbols that can be used in mandala. Tattva is a Sanskrit word meaning 'thatness', 'principle', 'reality' or 'truth'. In Hindu tantrism there are five (/'tʌtvəs/) tattvas creating global energy cycles of tides, which are tied to the lunar lunar tides and how they influence daily life. As well as the more subtle "tides" that are observed and recognized by Buddhist tradition that move through the universe and flow through and alternate at different times. This system of five tatras were also adapted by the Golden Dawn, an organization devoted to the study and practice of the occult, metaphysics, and paranormal activities during the late 19th and early 20th centuries.

"Every tree, every plant, has a spirit. People say that a plant has no mind. I tell them that a plant is alive and conscious. ... there is a spirit in it that is conscious that sees everything, which is the soul of the plant, its essence, what makes it alive."
---*Pablo Cesar Amaringo*

Pablo Cesar Amaringo Shuña was a Peruvian artist, renowned for his intricate, colorful depictions of his visions from drinking the entheogenic plant brew ayahuasca. Ayahuasca is a shamanic tool, very sacred, however a Schedule 1 hallucinatory drug. The parts of this plant medicine that I want to focus in are the benefits that can be reproduced with aromatherapy without the hallucinations and phase distortions, and within the law for those that are not a Shamanic practitioner. It is very sedative, opens one up to possibilities and broadening vision, increases the likelihood of embracing a magical way of thinking. Michael Pollan says that we are not evolving our plants, but rather the plants are evolving us. Vibrational aromatherapy deals primarily with the energetic qualities and application of essential oils which can involve a variety of energy healing modalities.

As Aromatherapists, we seek to bring harmony to the client, not treat the disease, knowing that belief plays a major role in certain bodily ailments.

Dr. Theresa Dale pioneered the first homeopathic formulas, according to the Fibonacci Numerical Sequence, which is based on one similar frequency being attracted to another similar frequency. Sounds similar to what we all know as universal energy. Have you ever used your body as an antenna to facilitate receiving and transmission of universal energy?

Would you be surprised to know that we are more like plants beyond our energy fields, beyond our defense systems, but in our very structure? Have you ever looked at the geometric structure found in the very bones that form our body's skeleton? What about how the navel divides the length of the body from head to toe at the Golden Section, the brow divides the face from the peak of the skull to the bottom of the chin, and the bottom of the nose marks the same division between the chin and brow?

The Fibonacci sequence was first recognized by the Indian Mathematician, Pingala who lived approximately 300 BCE to 200 BCE. The Fibonacci Series gets its name from Leonardo Fibonacci, who lived in the twelfth century. The Fibonacci sequence is a series of numbers in which each number is the sum of the two preceding numbers. Fibonacci Numerical Sequence is considered Sacred Geometry. This idea involves sacred universal patterns used in the design of everything in our reality, most often seen in sacred architecture and sacred art.

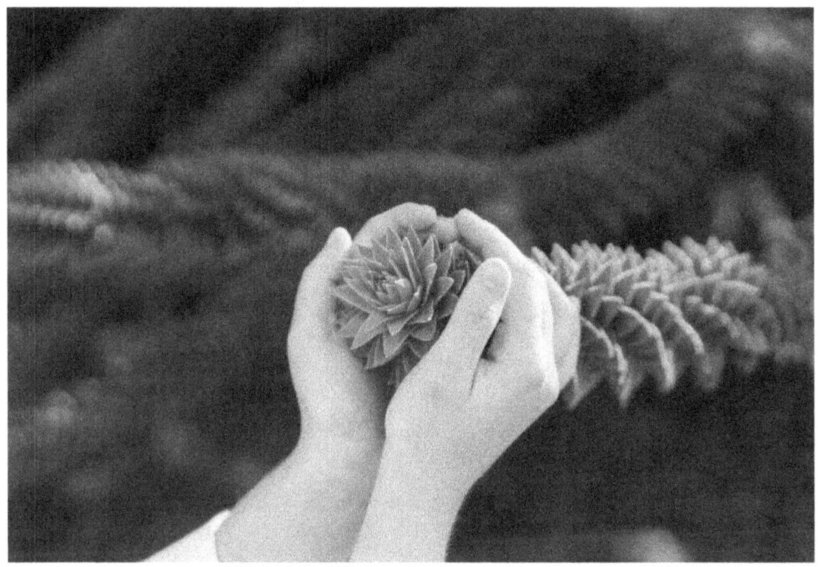

We find real world examples of the Fibonacci Series throughout the plant kingdom. Many plants that branch outwards towards the sun do so in branches equal to Fibonacci numbers, and florets on a cauliflowers, fruitlets on a pineapple, seeds on a sunflower, they all spiral outwards in a Fibonacci series. Plants can grow new cells in spirals, such as the pattern of seeds in the sunflower. The spiral happens naturally because each new cell is formed after a turn. New cell, then turn, another new cell, then turn, another new cell, then turn.

Leaves, branches and petals can grow in spirals, too. This is called Phi in Plant Forms or the Golden Ratio. Beyond being merely aesthetic, this spiral growth means that each leaf receives the maximum amount of sunlight to assist in photosynthesis. This Golden Ratio allows for a plant to retain its energy. Spiral galaxies also follow the familiar Fibonacci pattern. This is Sacred Geometry.

And it's not just in plants, and animals, hurricanes and the universe... but it's in us from our hands to the uterus. This connection has not been well explored in the human biology. Recent work at Florida International University at the Herbert Wertheim College of Medicine has begun to explore the understanding of such phenomenon documented at several different scales and systems in the human anatomy and physiology ranging from orthopedics, dentistry, the spiral of the human ear, the cardiovascular system and the human genome. Perhaps this amazing functionality in nature suggests its importance as a fundamental characteristic of the Universe, and why we are deeply connection to it all.

8

CHAKRA BALANCE

Just like the sacred geometry, we come to the number 8. Kundalini works with eight main chakras. The Root Chakra, the Lower Abdominal Chakra or Sacral Chakra, the Navel Chakra or Solar Plexus, the Heart Chakra, the Throat Chakra, and the widely known Eyebrow Chakra (also known as the Third Eye). There is also the Moon Chakra which is generally unrecognized but resides at the tip of your head on the back just under where most people have a cowlick. I've heard a belief that if you have two cowlicks at the back of your head, you have two energy centers. Only one modality that I have practiced recognizes the energy of this moon chakra by pulling energy into the session using a funnel that connects the knowledge or power point of electromagnetic energy connections, and the third eye. As well it this modality uses energy as a funnel and connector of energy channels for both restructuring energy and opening the upper chakras to allow the flow of energy through and out. And finally of course we have the Crown Chakra.

What is energy? Is energy about receiving, or manifesting or abundance? Let's talk about what receiving really means. To receive is simply to connect with energy. I can hand you a paper and you would receive it. Simple, just like that tangible paper, spiritual or abundant, or say manifested energy is no less real than any other energy, like electricity for example, but is vastly more important and easier to connect with. When you talk about spiritual energy, we call it prana or "universal life force" or "ki" (pronounced key which I find to be very interesting) and it is carried by pure love. This is something I have always believed in. I found it amazing when the Medical Medium said that God was the highest power, which is called, Love. So that higher energy is always love. In the English language 'heal' and 'holy' come from the same root. So love is an essential in our wellness energy.

I believe our bodies were built with that universal template of giving and receiving to elevate and enlighten our amazing infinite beings while we are in this life. Our bodies are this magical machine of cells that are giving and receiving throughout the day, even when we aren't aware of it. In fact when you hug someone it's not just that hormonal joy that you receive, but it's a microbiome based energy exchange that takes place as our microbiome are not just confined to our inner cells. Your microbiome is energy because as you'll soon find out, your immune system is energy. Everything about us is about giving and receiving energy. Everything about everything is energy. How does that feel?

We were made for this!! And not just receiving one bit of energy at one time. We have so many receptors that we are like those receptor cells waiting for the magnitude of peptides swirling about the universe. You may have been drawn to something like these for many years and felt that it is time to jump into it, even if it meant leaving that which has provided well for you. That feeling is called awareness. You may also feel like an imposter when you acknowledge energy, and that is called judgement. Now you are aware of your judgements and that makes it okay because as you feel it, you won't have any doubts at all about being and energy body, and soon you will release the judgements and just be. Deep within the spiritual center within your being is a this voice telling you that you are a vast expansive being … beyond anything you have imagined. That feeling, that awareness is what I want you to connect to. You are more than just a physical body, you are so much more. When we tune into what our body is asking for, it is actually tuning into the connection this minute physical being has to the forces around it.

We start with this discussion about Energy because it opens up all of the self-doubt in us, which gives you a way to release it, and then to help others. You can create with energy, you can heal with energy, you can believe in being energy and it can bring you joy like you have never experienced. This is all because you are energy. I am so glad you felt a calling or nudge to take this course, and when you follow your heart, you will realize what this possibility is offering you. We're going to first learn about this energy, and what it is before moving on.

Energy awareness…we sense it as a feeling. Sometimes it is a chill, or a cough, or a tingle. Awareness is a perception of energies, around us, in others, connections, perspectives and thus knowing. In order to be in awareness, you must be open to receiving energy. It's as gentle as taking a child's hand. Receiving is an energy transmission just like cell signaling, which sometimes happens within the cell itself.

I knew what energy was even when I was just teeny tiny, like some of you may have been aware of. Personally I have always been intuitive, and believe that it doesn't mean I am special. I think we all have the same powers of awareness available to us because we are all similar energy bodies. Energy bodies are not gender, or race, or blood types. When we become aware of this we can tap into our energy, and the energy from anywhere which allows us to pull energy when we need it.

How would you like to pull energy when you need extra to inspire, connect, or achieve something in the most authentic way? Energy is aligned to your purpose driven desire, even if it doesn't come to you in the way you think it will. That is where our judgement comes into play. Is this good work? Do you believe only Good will bring Joy. Only Good will bring nourishment. Only Good will bring that which you desire. Fill in the blank...It is that template of judgement. Belief in good and bad that creates this space where we block our ability to ignite our own source. I choose. That's the secret. You can choose good, you can choose joy, you can choose belief, you can choose something different. That is the real secret. Go there... and the rest will follow.

Ki remember is that universal life force energy that flows through each and every one of us, into everything and beyond. Think of Ki as a universal ocean that we all swim in. All things in the universe and out to the edges that are never ending in our physical and energetic world. We are energy beings. 99.999999% of your body is empty physical space but filled with energy. Our belief that we are these solid beings of matter is quite untrue. Ancient Rishis in India, who are regarded as "seers" or "sages", used intense meditation (tapas) thousands of years ago and realized the supreme truth and eternal knowledge, of our energetic bodies. Socrates, the teacher of Plato in Ancient Greece, also determined that energy, or soul, is separate from matter. He realized that the universe is made of a pure energy that was here before man and other material things like the earth came along.

Socrates believed in questioning everything. Questions give us awareness to the Ki around us.

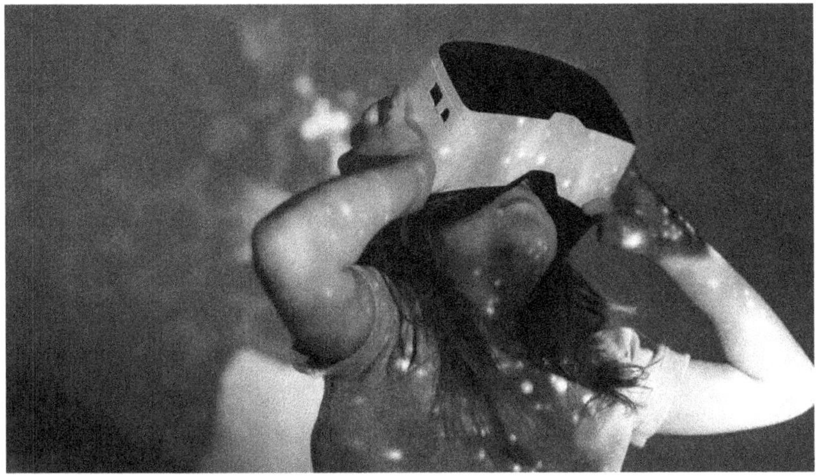

So if we aren't just matter (If we use quantum physics to look deep into the workings of the atom, we see that there is nothing there – just energy waves). Consider yourself instead to be made up of these energy waves of miniature tornadoes, which emit waves of electrical energy at all times in all directions. This has been scientifically measured, and thus we and the universe are just made up of energy.

As energetic bodies we continuously give off, and absorb, light and other energies, all the time. Giving and receiving even when we sleep. What is light? Light is this electric field connected to a magnetic field just flying through the energy cosmos. It's those energy wave receptors we call eyes that make light something special, and it is a chemical change that creates colors within the brain. Every cell in the body has its atoms lined up in such a way that it has a negative and a positive voltage, inside and outside. We are positivity and negativity in all moments. When they've measured your cells, each cell has 1.4

volts of energy – not much, but when you multiply by the number of cells in your body (50 trillion) you get a total voltage of 700 trillion volts of electricity in your body. Simply amazing!

If the body is mostly energy, it's no wonder that the energy soul is so easily considered to be the body. This duality is what creates such confusion in our daily living. Your atoms of energy each have their own distinct frequency, or vibration. When we choose we allow different atomic waves to meet up. These energies either meet in sync, creating a constructive or harmonious effect, or they meet out of sync, creating a destructive effect in which they annul each other. When we choose harmony we get harmony. When we choose discord we get disease and instability.

Our energy being isn't trapped inside of our bodies. People that are very in tune to our energy can see and read auras that are very near what appears to be our physical body. Your complex energy systems include what we call the Aura, our Chakras & the Meridian channels of the body. The Aura is believed to be similar electromagnetic mini-tornadoes just like the atoms that make up our body. The lower aura frequencies are connected to what we visualize as our metabolism and circulation. The higher frequencies then are what we visualize as our conscious and subconscious minds. Higher vibrations are related to your emotions, and are conveyed to others in what they see as our personality. Lower vibration disruptions can create tiredness, physical illness, an overall feeling of pain. Because auras are just energy, everything you see around you has an aura. There are those that are so tuned in that they see all of these colorful layers of energy. When they see an aura it is similar to what an energy healer may see when they are working on another person or themselves.

Auras change based on energy, and emotions are energy. In biochemistry and pharmacology, a receptor is a protein molecule that receives chemical signals from outside the cell, which could be from our own Aura or the energy exchange it has had with other auras around us. It creates a chemical signal like our eyes seeing light and our brain turning that light into the color green. These energetic chemical signals then binds to a receptor, causing some form of cellular/tissue response, what we call the change in the electrical activity of the cells. This is actively happening all of the time, and with many, many receptors.

We have a Vitamin D receptor present in most tissues and cells in the body, which was created to maintain the proper balance of several minerals in the body. When you sit in the sun, the rays create a chemical reaction that becomes pre-vitamin D. Pre-vitamin D spontaneously changes into the vitamin D we need. The receptor binds to that form to do some amazing things. The T-cells (which must be some amazing energy to do what they do) are the heroes of our immune system. They signal to the Vitamin D receptor to seek out the vitamin D from the bloodstream because these T-cells require Vitamin D to mobilize and fight. The initial energy exchange between the Sun's energy and our Aura is just one example of the importance of our energy and vibrations. If the body is minute molecules and we energy beings are energy atoms, it's important to understand that a chemical bond takes place between atoms in a molecule to create stability for all of the involved atoms. Just like the Vitamin D exchange, I like to think of our auras as the messenger to the physical body. They related the energies, and then the body uses them. This doesn't always happen the way we want it to, which is why understanding you can choose different energy is so important.

The belief currently is that the physical body has between four to seven layers of auras. They call the first layer the Ethereal Body which is just a layer of protection for the physical elements. This layer of the aura is where our chakras live. There is a belief that there is an energy cord that connects our innermost aura through our chakras into the Meridians, and that disconnect is what happens when we separate from our body to become simply energy in the afterlife. When I received my Karuna Ki Reiki Master attunement I saw the birth of my energy body, and it was quite powerful. I saw my father, God, as well, as I peered out around him to watch as he created everything that we see in this Universe. Our aura is the soul part of our energy, in my own personal experience.

The Astral body of our Aura is the part that exists in both the Heavenly Energy Plane, and the reality of our physical existence. It is that second layer. Some cultures believe that there are another five parts of the Astral Body called the skandhas. These are the physical body matter, the four elements of earth, air, water and fire; our emotions, our senses, the spark of our mental formations and our conscious awareness. This is why I believe that the Emotion Body and the Astral Body is the same layer of our energy being. Others may separate them where the Emotion Body is hosting the other five parts, and then the Astral Body. However, my personal belief is that they are all together and the same. The astral part of our aura, being part in this dimension of reality and part in the energy of all dimensions, is still influenced enough by reality, and feelings, to buy into this belief that we are not energy, that we are completely physical, and do not have the choices to create everything we desire. When we sleep it is far easier to connect to the Astral Plane, and that is where we often have those higher vibrational experiences. Intention lives in the astral layer of our Aura.

When you are attuned in Reiki it does not occur in the classroom, rather the knowledge is transferred from the Master to the recipient on the Astral Plane. When we reach the attunement time, remember that it's just energy, because thought or knowledge can be measured as energy.

As well, Karmic residue is carried in the Astral body. That is why it can be so easily cleared if we so desire to do it. We can choose to keep the energetic imprints and memories from our past lives with us, and often we do. Beyond our own karmic implants we often take on energies that are not ours. Such as the energies from Entities that do not have a body connection, as you do now. Buddhists believe that an entity is but an evolving consciousness, whose quality had been conditioned by karma. Releasing that energy of collective consciousness is one of most essential items you can do in this reality, in order to unburden your family and future family. There is a lot that can take place in the Astral Body, and those that work in shamanism are working through the astral body of all energies of plants, animals, and Entities. It is awareness that I think you may now be open to seeing.

The next layer is called our Mental Body. This is where the seed of consciousness was embedded into our existence. The mental body is where we take the knowledge energy and convert it into truth. Memories live in the initial layer of the Mental Body. It is the moments of Deja Vu that lives in our mental layer to tell us a little something is out there for you to be aware of. The electrical disturbance right before a seizure or a migraine is a part of the connection that this mental body has to our physical reactions. We only see it as a smash of colors before the moment of reality. I believe that there is something those people that deal with seizures, or migraines, are very closely connected to, and yet unable to be aware of. Some studies in China have also indicated that acupuncture could be beneficial for epilepsy, and I hope that they really start to bring quantum physics and Bio-Energy into the western medical arena very soon.

In our mental body whatever thoughts or emotions we choose, the energies vibrate at a certain frequency that is drawn to and attracts elements that vibrate at the same frequency. We want tornadoes that are just like ours. Coherence analysis is used to measure energy in our brain's networks. Where I believe that Reiki works through our Astral Body, I also believe that when we are working with specific points on our head, the work happens in our Mental Body. A recent study written up in the Energy Psychology Journal proved that treatment with a modality called Access Bars was associated with a significant decrease in the severity of symptoms of anxiety and depression and an increase in EEG coherence. So mind over matter, is exactly what we see happening in this layer of our aura. Some people believe that the Mental Body layer comes before the Astral Body; however this is what I feel.

The Spiritual Body Aura layer is where all of the truth lies. It is where the defined energies of what I often call your Soul Purpose lives. When you ask "truth" to define, clear or create and alternative awareness for you, this is where it happens. The current notion is that there are three layers of the spiritual aura. The first is the Etheric Template Body. This is where we seek to look past what we believe to be reality, and what it really is. This is where you can see and speak the truth, and where the energy flows to release what you are clearing away. When you think of your image, it is within the Etheric Template layer. It is exactly what it sounds like, your true self. You are not what you see in the mirror, which is why you may feel like your image is distorted when you look at your body in a mirror. Connecting to the energy in this layer will allow you to morph your physical body through the energetic work. I believe that the verbal clearings happen here, which is why the body can so easily just redefine the way it wants its energy to appear.

The second layer of the Spiritual Body is where wisdom comes from. Since energy is just energy, it is the truth bomb. All of our intuitive nature comes from the connection we have with this layer of our aura. When you are doing energy work and feel that third eye opening and become connected to the white light, you are working in your Spiritual body in this layer. Choice and awareness are open here, and everywhere you know, really know, is just energetic reactions from these spun energies of light. It is often related to indigo or violet. Violet energy waves have the shortest wavelength of the visible light spectrum, and they carry the most energy. That's why when you activate your third eye you will start seeing indigo or violet, or when you are very intuitive, or doing energy work like a Reiki or Bars session you will see a lot of this color.

Of course the third layer of the Spiritual Body is our Ketheric Template Body which is your spiritual purpose. If you believe that you had a choice in this life, and the parents you have, that is all energy from what they also call the Ketheric Body. This is where your Light Body lives. It is where you know that you are energy, that you have a higher calling, and it's all pure. Pure white light is all of it, because it has all of the energy colors from red, orange, yellow, green, blue, and violet all spread out. Although this white energy is often only felt or realized during energy and intuitive work, it can be seen by the most aware when they look at your aura. Some will also see a gold color in this layer, or a pink, brown, black, grey or twinkling silver in this aura field. These have to do with what is called Spiritual Alchemy, or transforming our self into the purest form possible. Being the outer edge of the aura it is the link to all of the universal energy, all higher sources, even God. The Ketheric Template Body is where Compassion relays truth.

Consider yourself instead to be made up of these energy waves of miniature tornadoes, which emit waves of electrical energy at all times in all directions. This has been scientifically measured, and thus we and the universe are just made up of energy.

Simple aura cleansing can be supported as well through the daily practices of smudging, mineral bathing or Earthing, which is placing your bare feet or skin in contact with the earth to take free electrons into the body.

If our Auras are connected to our Chakras, it's easy to see how having our chakras aligned and open to receiving is so important. When we work with Reiki and other similar energy modalities we are working through the blocks in the chakra energy field. Most of us look at the Chakra system as a system of 7 points, and so I will address those first. Each Auric body has its own set of seven major Chakras. These seven Chakras absorb energy-informational particles of different frequencies through the auras. These seven chakras are the root, sacral, solar plexus, heart, throat, third eye and crown. These are what we call three dimensional chakras. These connect the aura or energy body to the physical body, although they do not reside in any physical manner. Each chakra, however, does have a connection to our endocrine system and will influence it.

The Root Chakra is our grounding chakra that connects us to our Earth Life. Any considerations you have with being here on Earth are in this chakra. This chakra is associated with the Adrenal cortex glands, and as such influences physical energy, grounding and self-preservation. People dealing with physical imbalances, frequently getting sick, fatigue, lower back pain, feel cold, having emotional feeling of being unsafe, or unloved. These all connect to the adrenal glands and the root chakra. As well another interesting connection is a spacey feeling where you just let go of something. I dealt with severe adrenal fatigue for a very long time, and realized that I was choosing to make things disappear in order to have more difficulty in my life. Awareness to these types of aha moments will be very helpful. The root chakra is often associated with the color Red. I find that when I am physically active and I am doing something in nature, this chakra is much more in tune. And then my adrenals function so much better. Connected to memory, time and space.

The Sacral Chakra is what we call the polarity chakra, as in electronic signaling. That transformation of our mind when we meditate starts with the hypothalamus, which is the endocrine connection to our sacral chakra. It responds to both internal and external signals. Doesn't it make sense that being able to react appropriately to stress, would in turn help to align our root? No wonder this chakra is next in line. It has been called the cruise control button for the limbic system. That means it regulates the speed of your heartbeat, and many other metabolic functions. We often see the color orange associated with this chakra. Another gland connected to this chakra is the leydig gland. This relatively unknown gland is normally a pea-sized gland located in the lower abdomen along the centerline of our body, and becomes inactive in most people around age 20. It is located more or less halfway between the umbilicus or belly button and the penis in men or the vagina in women. It is about 1 inch inside the body, nearer the front of the body. The gland serves as an anchor point for the etheric body, and when active secretes chemicals that assist with spiritual development. One of the most important functions of the hypothalamus is to link the nervous system to the endocrine system via the pituitary gland, as they are attached. Our third eye is connected to the pituitary gland, and so it makes sense that all of these glands are connected. Connected to reason.

The Solar Plexus Chakra is connected to both Pancreatic and Adrenal Glands. These two glands do work very closely together and the adrenal glands straddle two chakras rather than one. The pancreas aids in digestion, and helps control the levels of energy in the blood. So you will see this chakra associated with yellow. If you think about the digestive system being the core of everything in our bodies, it is no wonder this area is associated with so many physical imbalances of the digestive body, and then also the connected microbiome axis issues, from memory and beyond. Connected as well to willpower.

The Heart Chakra is truly special. When I am working intuitively the energy flows out to the individual through my heart chakra. The thymus gland they say holds the key to aging. It is the main organ of our lymphatic system, and has the primary function of developing our T-cells. Autoimmune illnesses are when the body determines its own cells to problems and sends the T-cells to attack them. Researchers suspect that autoimmune processes are a factor in heart disease. This gland is only active until puberty. After puberty, it starts slowly shrinking and becomes replaced by fat. Perhaps stimulation of this gland will be the key to aging and disease in the future. Of course the Heart Chakra also controls our hearts. It's a very emotion driven chakra, and has a lot to do with how we accept ourselves. It is often connected with the color green, and I find this fitting because nature can always boost my mood. Our heart is in charge. They now say we have our regular brain, our gut brain and our heart brain. The heart brain doesn't do as much as the regular brain, however it does tell it what to do. Connected to direct cognition.

The Throat Chakra is all about how we communicate and express ourselves. Also connected to that very in line with how we use our free will. This chakra is connected with the thyroid gland, and as such seems fitting that so many people I know with thyroid issues have had moments of not having a voice. Not surprising the throat chakra can be connected to many hormonal disorders, and a lot of mood functions. The color of the throat chakra is blue, and is often the first auric color people will see. So it's no wonder that our throat chakra is connected to the ability for telepathy and intuitive hearing, which is also called clairaudience. I can't say that I hear spirits, yet. I have clairvoyance which means I can see things in dreams, or see images when I close my eyes. My daughter laughs that my most used sentence is "I see". I also have clairsentience which is what empaths are, and means clear feeling. I also have claircognizance which is clear knowing. I just know things.

Recently I had someone message me asking about a jawbone infection. I knew exactly what was causing it. I have heard that singing helps the throat chakra, and I find this amazing because it also stimulates the vagus nerve. All of our chakras connect from the brain and the spine, via our vagus nerve to these glands. When you hear someone talk about kundalini awakening, it seems like they were talking about the vagus nerve. The Kundalini snake coils three times as it travels up the spine, just as the vagus nerve does. How great is it that your throat chakra can awaken and stimulate everything else in your seven chakras?

Your voice is essential to find so that you can create your own awakening. Connected to divine love. Maybe that is why you should not speak when you have nothing good to say.

The Third Eye is generally very open in those that have all of these gifts I have talked about because it is your inner sight, spiritual visions. Remember that it is associated with the indigo color, and the pituitary gland which is called the master gland. This gland contains the nerve endings of neurons from the hypothalamus, like oxytocin, where it is stored until it needs to be released into the bloodstream. The hormones of the pituitary gland send signals to all of these other endocrine glands to stimulate or inhibit their own hormone production. It's said the best way to strengthen your pituitary gland is to meditate. This third eye is considered a portal for universal energies. Connect to divine sight.

I have a lot of people ask me about opening their third eye. They are often energy healers, and want to be able to offer more. The crown chakra, which is really the true gate to the higher vibration energies, is associated with the pineal gland. The formation of crystals (called calcification) and cysts is what I have learned is related to an iodine deficiency. Fluoride can displace iodine, and in highly fluoride areas, you often see low iodine as well. Calcification is the biggest problem for the pineal gland since fluoride accumulates in the pineal gland and forms those phosphate crystals. So as your pineal gland hardens, you also get less melatonin. So it's a cycle of issues that do not work well for opening or activating your third eye.

The Crown Chakra is connected to all things illuminating, and is connected to several other chakras. Leader of the basic chakra system, and connected to our identity, sense of meaning, and all of the emotions of loss in those areas. The crown chakra can become very overactive when you are downloading a lot of spiritual energy and information. Symptoms can include sensitivity to light, dizziness, and lack of caring, brain fog or confusion. The crown relies on us to eat well in order to restore balance to our entire chakra system. Energy work, slow moving wellness like Tai Chi and crystal work can all help rebalance this chakra and in such, rebalance your chakra system. Understanding how connected the Crown and the Third eye are may help you understand why the Crown chakra is often related to poor sleep and brain dysfunction. As a gorgeous violet color, it was the first color I can remember experiencing after a spark of white during my first Reiki attunement.

The Sanskrit word, kundalini, means coiled, like a snake. Kundalini energy is not recognized by medical science, much like plant medicine of all holistic modalities. Kundalini is said to rise up from the Root Chakra, and via spirals it moves through the spine and all of the different Chakras reaching the top of the crown. This progress leads to different levels of awakening, and a transformation of consciousness. It is important to remember that kundalini energy does not spiral through our physical body, but your etheric or subtle body. Chakra grids, visualizing grid patterns, our Pineal Gland… all of this has to do with that sacred geometry and raising your Kundalini energy. In fact your pineal gland is a sacred geometric shape, and shaped like a pinecone. There are many ways to use energy modalities to help your kundalini energy along, as well as balance the chakras.

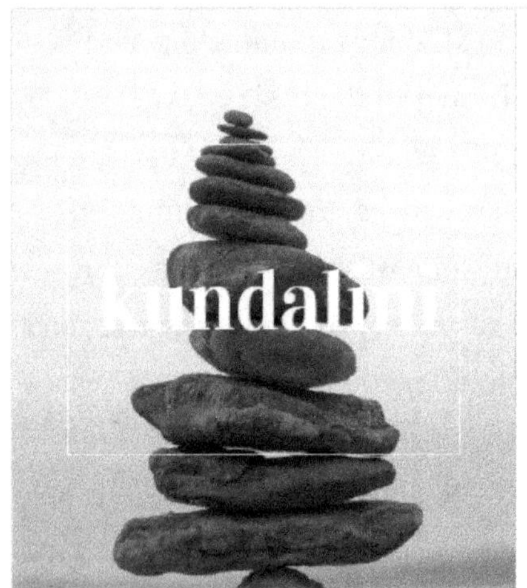

Considered to the biological third eye, it receives the highest percentage of blood flow of any other area of the body other than the kidneys. The Bible itself alludes to pinecones and the Pineal Gland on several occasions, sometimes quite specifically. Beginning in Genesis, Jacob wrestles all night with God, and is commanded to change his name to Israel. The bible then purports the following:

And Jacob called the name of the place Peniel: *"For I have seen God face to face, and my life is preserved. And as he passed over Peniel the sun rose upon him.*

Many Bible readers may not know that the translation of the word "Peniel" means "Face of God".

What I find most interesting is that in the brain structure, the pineal gland is unpaired. Your only one pineal gland, sits right on the midline of the brain. Melatonin is released by the pineal gland. The amount of melatonin found in spinal fluid is much higher than the amount in our bloodstream, and it controls our circadian rhythm. Think about the fact that melatonin is secreted throughout the night with the absence of light, while yoga science states our 3rd eye awakening brings forth the light of a thousand moons. The amount of melatonin found in spinal fluid is much higher than the amount in our bloodstream. Though not paired up in the brain, the structure of the retina and pineal gland are very similar, the theory is that the pineal gland consists of a variety of genes that are only expressed in the eye; thus, the pineal gland has photoreceptors and a complete system for optical transduction. That would mean there is a light-communication highway to the pineal gland, but only if we see it. Due to chemicals in our world, the pineal gland is often calcified.

Dr. Dr. Edward Group says, "Fluoride accumulates in the pineal gland more than any other organ and leads to the formation of phosphate crystals. As your pineal gland hardens due to the crystal production, less melatonin is produced and regulation of your wake-sleep cycle gets disturbed." In medical studies, pineal gland calcification has been proposed to play a role in the pathogenesis of Alzheimer disease, after using cone-beam computed tomography scans of patients referred for dental implant therapy who could possibly be a vulnerable group for this condition. However calcification of the pineal gland is typical in young adults, and has been observed in children as young as two years old. Using Cedarwood, Frankincense and Sandalwood can be very therapeutic for the third eye.

Chakra in Sanskrit is roughly translated to "wheel", and refers to the chakras perceived vortex of rotating geometric energy. Your chakra is believed to be spherical in shape, like the sacred geometry shapes throughout the universe. They expand out in all three dimensional directions in a spiral motion, with a radius extending out for hundreds of kilometers. They spin in both clockwise and counterclockwise directions, interacting with the major and minor chakras through the earth's energy field. Some of the top intersecting connections are believed to be found in the Himalayas, the Peruvian Inca territories and in Sedona, Arizona. In the Kabbalah every circle is aligned with one chakra. The flower of life is the 13 dimensions or dimensional systems of consciousness, the seed of life is our chakras, and the Seed of life inside the fruit of life is the merging of the dimensions within our chakra system together they create the flower of Life.

Aromatherapy can help open each energy chakra of our body. You can use essential oils with meditation, energy work, while visualizing, working with a singing bowls; the list goes on and on.

When working with the Root Chakra, balancing, grounded, safe and happy oils will help with clearing imbalance. Cedarwood, Myrrh, Patchouli and Vetiver are my favorites. Thyme and Ylang Ylang can also be helpful.

The Lower Abdominal Chakra oils help us move, and get our groove back, and are also very uplifting. Ylang Ylang is a good crossover oil and is Patchouli. You can also balance with Cardamom, Orange, Clary Sage, Sandalwood and Bergamot.

When you feel incomplete, lack confidence or patience, are inflexible and just desire a calm inner being, the Navel Centre needs a bit of balance restored. Again, Ylang Ylang is a wonderful balancing oil for those lower chakras, as is Cedarwood and Sandalwood. I also love some of the spicy oils like Cinnamon, Black Pepper to increase willpower, and Clove. Although Spearmint, Coriander, Ginger,

Rosemary, Tangerine, Grapefruit, and Lemongrass are all amazing oils to use for this area. Are you seeing a theme there? I also find that diffusing Cypress, Juniper or Vetiver is very supportive for our Solar Plexus instability.

The Heart Chakra is so easily imbalanced when we are not in awareness of truth. You feel less contented, unhappy, unloved, and unable to give love, unable to receive, and give. You can lose all that you feel purposeful about, and all that is compassionate. Ylang Ylang and Sandalwood jump out again as wonderfully balancing heart oils. Also the citrus bunch is all there with Orange, Lemon, Tangerine, or Bergamot. One of my favorite stress control blends includes Lemon, Copaiba, Cedarwood, Pine, Neroli, Lavandin, Lime and True Lavender. Of course True Lavender is a wonderful balance for the heart, as is Rose, Jasmine and Cypress.

The Throat Chakra is one that I see a lot in my practice. People not speaking their truth, people not opening up and vocalizing their needs. But besides lacking the ability to communicate expressively, the throat chakra also impacts our ability to listen to others, share our honestly with them, and be open to taking criticism. It's also where patience gets lost. This is an area where I really had to work to balance. My favorite oil for balance here is Basil. I also love Bergamot, Cypress, Peppermint and Spearmint, and Roman Chamomile. Roman Chamomile also helps open the crown so that you can have the knowledge you desire to share.

The pineal or Eyebrow Chakra obviously is out of balance when you can't hit your intuition no matter what you do. You are impulsive, lack common sense, are stuck in old memories, or lose an ability to remember, become over analytical, and lacking faith. You can be very judgmental of others and yourself when out of balance in your third eye. And forget sleep when you aren't producing enough melatonin, and when you do sleep your dreams aren't what you desire. Frankincense is my go to oil for this area, but I love Vetiver, Rosemary, Sandalwood, Cypress, Clary Sage, Juniper, Helichrysum, Patchouli, and for deeply rooted pain, Marjoram.

When your Moon Chakra is out of balance, you will have a physical and mental fatigue. It can impact your ability to see what is happening; feel out of harmony, lack clarity and balance. Hyperactive and nervous? Struggling with your psychic and spiritual health? This is the chakra with the most oomph for gaining vitality. Similar to the oils for the Eyebrow Centre, the Moon Centre offers some amazing energy, although it often sleeps. When it is awakened it really will begin to flow opening up streams of cosmic creativity. When struggling to sleep you can gently massage this chakra with soft circular movements, envisioning the geometric vibration as it opens up to harmony and quiet.

The Crown Chakra is everything for your universal energy downloads. Without balance in this center you can feel very unspiritual, lack purpose, lack God, or try to recreate yourself as God. There can be a lot of anger in this chakra, and a great fear of reaching the end, especially due to the lack of connection one feels to self, others and a higher power. All of the grounding oils are wonderful for this center like Frankincense, Vetiver, Cedarwood, Sandalwood, Vetiver, but also Helichrysum, Rose, Jasmine and Lavender.

Using aromatherapy with other modalities to balance your chakras can open up so many possibilities. The etheric body is linked to the base chakra, and so you can see why from the Crown to the Root chakra, everything matters.

I would like to ask you to stop before continuing on into the more advanced chakra knowledge and ground your system with my daily grounding ceremony. This video can be found on my YouTube channel https://youtu.be/bu0lkYHangI

Grounding is this process that helps our physical body to connect to surrounding energies, and can open you up to what we are going to move into next.

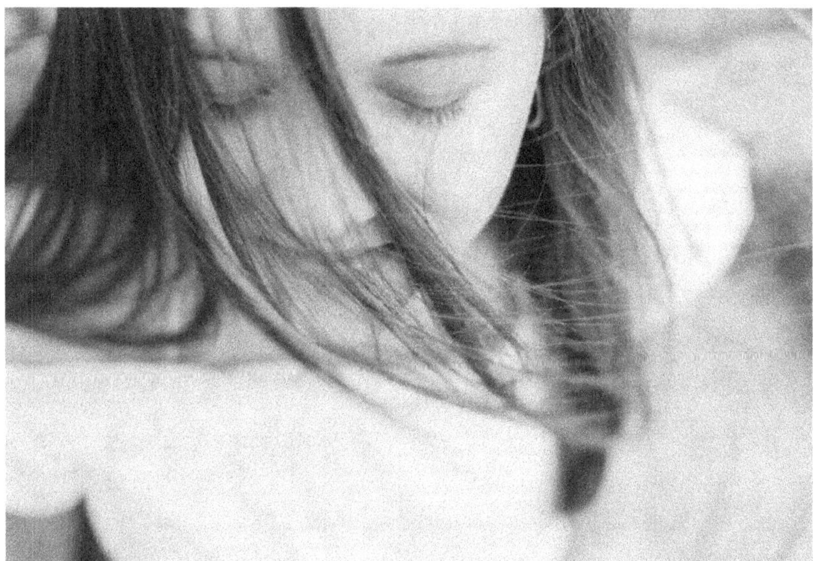

9

CHAKRA BALANCE ADVANCED

There are of course more than the eight chakras that I have already shared with you. How many do you think there are? Nine… ten… twelve??

There are actually 114 chakras in the body. When we practice the postures in Sun salutation, it is designed to impact all the vital chakras and open you up for energy reception throughout the day. Two of the 114 chakras are outside our own physiological framework. These are the points where the energy channels the body. These energy channels are called "nadis," and there are 72,000 in our body. Since we could never cover all of that in this course, we will lightly go beyond the eight that we have already discussed in order to understand and use chakra balancing in your aromatherapy practice.

Beyond the others, we are told that only 108 need actual work, and they will open up the other four. There is an energy channel that connects to all of the channels and chakras above and below that is placed at the top of our head. It is as if you just sliced off the top of your head. As energy healers we can create a crown around this, and pull energy up into those upper chakras and our energy source to open up to all of the knowledge and knowing available. The best example that I can give is to imagine cutting the top off of a head of garlic. It is that upper part that is this crown of connecting all of the bodies. Using energy modalities that work with this, you can open up all of the energy channels, and bring a unquantifiable awareness into your life.

'Hrit' which means he who dwells in the heart, is located between the solar plexus and the heart, just under the heart. This chakra has eight petals unlike the heart's twelve red petals, has gold petals and is as delicate as a lotus, and red as the morning sun. This chakra normally points downward, but should be raised upward when you are working on it. It is also called the root or bulb of bliss. When you look at Tibetan Buddhism, there is a similar chakra called the Fire Wheel. This is located above the heart and below the throat. The Hrit chakra absorbs energy from the sun, and this warms our energetic body, and all other chakras. Because of this it is sometimes called the Sun Chakra. If you wonder why vitamin D is so essential to our wellness, perhaps this is why. Using Ylang Ylang or Sandalwood essential oils will help balance and create an opening to work with this chakra.

Manas (which means mind) main chakra point is located between the navel and the heart, and is very linked to the third eye as it has an upper chakra point that is located below the third eye chakra. This has a channel of energy that runs between the two points. Perhaps this is why the microbiome is so tied into our brain. As a power energy this chakra has eight petals below and six petals above. This chakra is the filter between the pure energy and our chitta. Chitta is considered the "mind-stuff", which are the lower energies of emotions and ego. The chitta channel is centered in the heart, and yoga helps us to calm and release some of that chatter. Lavender has a calming effect as does

Orange, Vetiver, Frankincense, Cedarwood and Ylang Ylang. For those of you that are also massage therapists, massage opens up this energy channel for a more focused yet calm mind. No wonder we feel so amazing after a good massage.

The real Crown chakra is located far above our head, and has a lotus of 100 white petals. I call this the Nirvana Chakra, and it works at fine tuning the pure white energy that comes from the source to our being. I have seen sources that say that it is actually a thousand petalled lotus, which I wouldn't doubt at all being what it does for us. Imagine one thousand petals, arranged from right to left, in twenty layers, each containing fifty petals, and the arrangement of the petals giving the appearance of a bell. The lunar region is golden in color. Because of its aura of white light, it is often called the Halo chakra. Visually it looks like a starburst of energy, and I believe it is the energy that we draw when you see photos of angels with halos. This chakra is the supreme chakra in our consciousness development.

In between the Crown chakra and the Nirvana Chakra is a minor chakra called the Guru Chakra which is also called the "doorway filled with light". Ylang Ylang and Frankincense are wonderful essential aromas to use in connecting to the upper chakra energies. Guru is our higher knowledge and is often called the Seat of the Master. It is an upward facing 12 petalled lotus that guides the energy for our spiritual journey. Consider this where all of the soul's knowledge is available. This chakra is the connection to where our soul will access the path home when our physical body dies. This bridge chakra is essential to work on to gain brain development of knowledge.

Between your Eyebrow or Third Eye chakra and the Nirvana Chakra is the energy channel that controls breathing. We pass through our energy through this channel to reach the bridge chakra, and different possibilities.

If you were to draw a line from the Moon Chakra down to the middle of the base of the spine, you would connect the channel to the Alta Chakra, which is also called Alta Major. It sits centered on the medulla oblongata. This shows up as either a twelve petal lotus and red, or a sixty-four petal lotus and gleaming white. My intuition tells me that when working with Alta Major on the body, it will show up as 12 petals, and when working with the Alta Major in the etheric field it will show up as sixty-four petals.

When we have an energy block, it is often connected to this chakra point as it aligns with the Reticular Activating System which is a network of nerve pathways in the brainstem connecting the spinal cord, cerebrum, and cerebellum, and mediating the overall level of consciousness. You can access the RAS through a small band that runs across the base of your head. You can also use quartz to clear out energies in the Alta Major, or the RAS which will clear the connection from the upper energy points through the rest of the body, and your energy fields. Making sure we get enough minerals is essential for this chakra to balance and function properly. Minerals are required for conductors to fire between nerve synapses. Forms of mineral salts, brain tissue salts and homeopathic remedies can also be helpful, remembering to separate use of homeopathic treatments and aromatherapy.

The Alta Major chakra is often called the Mouth of God or Goddess, and opens your kundalini channel to multiple dimensions. It is considered to be a dimensional doorway. It is important to know this information when working through a time shift. Using oils that offer grace, strength and protection can be important for this chakra. The color of this chakra is very bright magenta. Working with Alta Major you can rewire your brain. This point has channels that connect to all of our considerations through all dimensions, realities, lifetimes, space, and of course all of our energy.

Bring connected to our medulla oblongata. The medulla oblongata is the part of the brain that helps regulate breathing, heart and blood vessel function, digestion, sneezing, and swallowing. It is said to have been formed from the original nucleus of energy at our current lifetime moment of conception.

Alta has a polarity connection to the third eye and the crown chakra. It allows the prana or life force to enter your body, and directs all of the incoming cosmic energy. When we are feeling a migraine energy stemming from this space, it's easy to imagine that there may be an imbalance in this chakra projecting all of the incoming energy through it and to all areas of the body that are blocked and unwell. Chiropractic manipulation or adjustment can bring great relief in this area.

This chakra is deeply connected to the implants that we have placed upon our being. An implant can be considered to be like an energetic virus. It is a tick that we allow to burrow deep into our energy that blocks the voice of our angels, inner knowing, and our Spirit guides. Behind the ear is where we then store these implants from all of our lifetimes unless we release them.

Energy implants can stretch out through the channels to any of your chakra points, and through Energy Medicine or many other alternative modalities, you can work with these areas that are stuck. Implants lower our vibrations, whereas meditation, whole foods, vibrations, sound and any energy work you may do, including aromatherapy, will rise up into higher vibrations and the higher energy source.

Is any wonder that this Alta Major is also the location of the connection to the central nervous system? Part of our central nervous system is that autonomic nervous system which is the director of our physical response to stress. The most common essential oils use to this system is Bergamot, Lavender, and Geranium, with my preference to Bergamot due to research I have seen. Fifty-four elementary school teachers from three different schools were enrolled in a study using Bergamot as aromatherapy diffusion. Aromatherapy was conducted once a week using an Ultrasonic Ionizer Aromatherapy Diffuser for aroma evaporation. 100% pure bergamot essential oil was used and diluted to 2%. Physiological parameters were recorded by an ANSWatch monitor, and each session was recorded for seven minutes. The average blood pressure and heart rate variability parameters were shown on the panel of ANSWatch monitor. After looking at the data the conclusion was that after two 10-minute aromatherapy sprays with Bergamot essential oil on elementary school teachers, the parasympathetic nervous system, one of three divisions of the autonomic nervous system, which stimulates the vagus channel, was enhanced and shown on corresponding physiological parameters. The teachers with moderate and high degrees of anxiety benefited more than the light anxiety group. Aromatherapy seems to drive autonomic nervous activity toward a balanced state.

We can help our parasympathetic nervous system in other ways. This includes deep breathing exercises, grounding into the here and now moments, relaxing our muscles through thought or physical manipulation, NLP, Heart Math training, binaural beats, meditation, cold therapy and slower moving exercises that are very thoughtful.

This chakra has roots reaching down through the spine, moving that kundalini energy into the root chakra where is disperses throughout the body and all of the energy branches and channels up to the crown chakra.

Imprints are what are left behind from an implant, as a knotted energy field. When you have done work to remove these implants, it still takes time for these knots to unbundle and release into the energy flow. It is in this space that aromatherapy can really do some amazing things to ease up a return to beliefs and doubts that you have cast on your life. Like a knot in a tree, the tree can continue to grow, but the knot sometimes remains. Knots which we consider to be blemishes in trees often cause lumps or holes within the trunk of the tree itself. These knots are usually caused by the natural growth of the tree, though the specific circumstances under which they form determines how they will appear. Knot hunters use saws to hack the knot off, giving the tree a fresh wound. How many times have you allowed others, or even yourself, to do the same?

Using fiercely healing oils where you feel a knot is forming, can help to release before it becomes a part of the landscape. Peppermint, Lavender, Frankincense, Juniper, Rosemary and Clove, along with the seldom used Turmeric Essential Oil are very powerful healer aromas for these imprinted knots. This imprint is also called samskara. When you feel that heart feeling as an empath, you are causing an implant to be created, and an imprint starts forming. Implants separate us from consciousness, and constrict our energy flow. Imprints cause pain in the body, pain in our thoughts, and pain on an emotional level. When pain happens, we start to focus inward on it, rather than outward toward the source.

Yogis believe that the journey of unsticking these imprints is our path. It is meant to help guide us in releasing all of the other things we think we need in life, and remove the attachments. Using energy, we can use electricity instead to begin to unravel these knots of energy, and open up the flow of receiving again.

Lower chakras that we will focus in on are also called Talas. These chakras run down the leg, and connect us to our base animal instincts. 100 million Americans suffer from chronic pain. Eastern cultures, have worked to help bring about harmonious attitudes and feelings via working with the physical body for thousands of years. Those short-circuited emotions become stuck in time in DNA passed from generation to generation. When researchers in Finland had people map out where they felt different emotions on their bodies, they found that the results were surprisingly consistent, even across different cultures. Misalignment of our body systems can happen through social conditioning, trauma or trauma-like experiences, and general, prolonged tension or anxiety; as well as from the electrical connection we have to the world around us, emotions we have brought with us from birth, past lives and parallel journeys. Empaths can absorb the emotions as well as physical pains.

Past life emotions are sometimes called karmic emotions. Even Freud assumed that the muscles of the body had something to do with storing the emotions of repression. Neuroscientist Antonio Damasio believes that each emotion activates a distinct set of body parts, and the mind's recognition of those patterns helps us consciously identify that emotion. Researchers in the UK found that applying lemon balm oil to the faces and arms of patients with severe dementia reduced their agitation by 35 percent. Using the emotion map can help you to start working on those emotions that are stuck in your physical body, and to keep a record of the essential oils that work well for you. Trauma that is transferred from the first generation of trauma survivors to the second and further generations of offspring of the survivors is called transgenerational transmission of trauma. It is interesting to see how all of this relates to the lower chakra systems.

The hips are where we often hold onto birth trauma and fear related to birth. The lower Atala Chakra is located in our hips and it is where fear resides. Along with fear, it is the storage ground for negative feelings and pent-up emotions, like promiscuity and lust, and emotions related to being in control. The essential oils Bergamot, Grapefruit, Lime, and Orange are all very helpful in releasing emotions stuck in the hips. You may also use Jasmine, Clary Sage, Rosemary, Marjoram or Sage to address your controlling fears. Smudging a palo santo stick is also a helpful aroma for the Atala Chakra.

Centered in our thighs are the emotions of blame, resentment, anger and betrayal. This space is where the lower chakra Vitala lives. The talas are brutally honest about how we feel. This center can create raging anger inside of us. You must increase feelings of safety through the use of Basil, Chamomile, Pine, Rosemary and Thyme. Also increasing joy using Bergamot, Grapefruit, Lime and Orange essential oils. Since the hip flexors are a group of muscles around the top of your thighs that connect your upper leg to your hip, addressing both

Atala and Vitala can be supportive in releasing the stuck energies connected to this group of muscles. Also use of boat pose and pigeon can bring up some strong emotions to the surface to address and offer an opening for expansive oils to work.

Your Sutala chakra point is located in the knees, and is a very restrictive energy space. Emotions tied to this resistance, lack, helplessness and envy can be stuck in our knees. This leads to a very combative nature. How many times are you saying, "I can't have" per day. It's important to remember that beyond this lower chakra point, every joint has their own chakras as well. Cypress is a magical oil for this chakra. As well, Sandalwood is always an amazing oil to move the most stagnant of emotions.

Roman Chamomile will unravel the emotions of anger, recklessness and lack. A great oil for aligning these three lower chakras to release these deep seeded emotions.

Talatala is often out of balance in young children and our aging parents where they are recklessly abandoning our guides, and making bad choices due to the emotions that are driven by confusion. As well this center fuels by the feeling of, "I've got mine, get lost and go get yours." Greed festers in this chakra that is centered in our calves. The first signs of imbalance can be felt with the unpleasant feelings from restless leg syndrome. Cypress, Coriander, Frankincense, Ginger, Lavender, Peppermint, Rosemary, Cedarwood and Spruce are all helpful to use with this lower chakra imbalance. Pairing with Chamomile or Pine will help you to feel more protected.

Emotions tied to how we feel about our parents get stored in the legs from the thighs through the knees and down though the calves.

Heavier energy right leg energy contains emotions from our connection to our Father, and the left leg is connected to our Mother. Releasing the energy from your thighs helps us to believe in ourselves, the knees will release the fear of change, and the lower leg will help you move toward your desired goals. All of these emotions get tied together, and so it's important that we don't stop our energy healing at just the root chakra. We are a whole body of energy, and a whole body of points that can create a blockage in the natural flow.

Rasatala of course then is the point in our ankles. How many have a lot of stagnation in the ankles? What is it about changing direction that you are unsure of? Where is your life feeling unbalanced? When we have stuck energy in our ankles we have put ourselves first. This is a very selfish energy that can be brought on by very intense fear, which often stems from emotional abuse. Emotions will cycle in the ankles causing everything else to slow down and get stuck along with it. It's a complex chakra because having stuck energy in this point doesn't mean you aren't being of service to your fellow man. It showcases that you are lacking true empathy, and have an underlying narcissistic behavior that others don't usually see until they are in the middle of your exploitive behavior. Also overly impulsive and can struggle with jumping into something before you consider the consequences. The mother of all essential oils for this lower chakra is Frankincense. Using this along with Cypress, Lemongrass, Geranium and Marjoram can help you consider others before yourself. As you start putting those relationships in your life back together, these energies will start to flow through the body with much more ease.

Our ankles are receptacles for all of the energies we are refusing to release, however our feet feel the need to do everything they can to support this body structure. Mahatala is the overall lower chakra that is aligned to our feet, tough Patala is the lower chakra of our soles. Reflexology is very helpful when used with essential oils to get energy moving from the feet. Mahatala has an emotional belief that you are karmically owed. This energy will bounce back and forth between the foot and the ankle for years when not addressed. Using Melissa, Geranium, Frankincense, Sandalwood, True Lavender, Lemon, Jasmine, Roman Chamomile, Bergamot, Ylang Ylang, Helichrysum and Rose can address this energy, and walk you through forgiveness. Without it the energy can turn very negative in the Patala chakra where revenge and hatred will fester and harden your energy body. Those with utter disrespect for other humans have very hard, unmoving energy in this lowest chakra point. Working with movement, essential oils, reflexology, energy healing, and grounding your being with a feeling of connecting to the highest powers can help bring back a sense of stability.

Our Meridians are the energy channels that flow within the body to acupoints where life force is accessible close to the surface of the skin. Through linking the meridian system to the chakra system in our lesson, it will make chakra balancing more profound. An understanding that our meridians give entry points to energy from the chakra points into the body system channels, and helps us to understand how all of this is tied together.

Recently scientists at Seoul National University confirmed the existence of meridians, which they refer to as our "primo-vascular system" or PVS. The PVS is a previously unacknowledged system that integrates the features of the cardiovascular, nervous, immune, and hormonal systems. It is connected to many biological processes like tissue regeneration, inflammation and cancer. They found the presence of these primo vessels in and around blood and lymph vessels, nerves, fascia, and in the brain and our spinal cord.

Your meridians are paired bilaterally, and named after the major organs in the body. The 12 major meridians in the body are: Bladder, Gallbladder, Heart, Kidney, Large Intestine, Liver, Lung, Pericardium, Small Intestine, Spleen, Stomach and the Triple Warmer. Research shows that both energy and blood flow through the meridians, and transmit information to the organs they are connected to. On a basic level it could be to release water, or lower your body temperature. With their sensitivity they can easily become blocked from any number of causes including a block within the chakras.

Traditional Chinese Medicine works to release energy to flow freely through the meridians using herbs, acupuncture, movement, food and more. The Stomach Meridian flows into the Spleen Meridian. The Heart Meridian flows into the Small Intestine Meridian. Your Bladder Meridian flows into the Kidney Meridian. The Pericardium Meridian flows into the Triple Warmer Meridian. The Gallbladder Meridian flows into the Liver Meridian. The Lung Meridian flows into the Large Intestine Meridian. There is a yin and yang pairing within our meridians that is both simplistic and beautiful.

If we look at the Auras, the Astral Body is where the skandhas is, which contains those Earth Elements of the subtle body. Similarly each Meridian is related to one of those elements. In order to rebalance those imbalances it is important in understanding how energy therapies or modalities impact our bodies. Think of it in this way.

YOUR 12 MERIDIAN PAIRS WORK IN FUNCTIONS

Liver and Gallbladder meridian = food and energy intake

Kidney and Bladder meridian = purification and hormone system

Heart and Small Intestine = adaptation and control

Lung and Large Intestine meridian = excretion

Stomach and Spleen meridian = digestion

Pericardium and Triple Warmer = circulation and protection

Stress is the primary reason our body's meridian system repeatedly becomes imbalanced. This results in health problems that won't go away after many attempts using traditional methods.

Many energy healing modalities work on rebalancing and releasing stuck energy in the meridians. A lot of energy workers can feel this energy, but haven't ever understood what they are feeling. When Ki touches old energies stuck in the consciousness or the body, it opens up the possibilities for new choices and paths. Recent studies confirm that meridians have many biophysical properties, including electric characteristics, thermal characteristics which make sense if you have worked with infrared therapy before, acoustic characteristics, optical characteristics, magnetic characteristics, isotopic characteristics and myoelectric characteristics.

Any imbalance in the meridians can create so many problems in balancing your chakras. So when we consider nutrients, hydration, harmony, relaxation, our microbiome and movement into the equation you can sense why a healthy body means more than you have been told. We require a healthy body in order to have a deep connection to energy. We require a practice of working with energy in order to have a healthy body. More balance, and that yin and yang energy polarity. Energy knows where to go, and we as energy healers we aren't healing, we are channeling energy in the same way that all of the subtle body has been created to do. When working with a Reiki Master they are working to seek out auras that the meridians are emitting.

There are many ways to balance and work on the subtle bodies. Smudging versus essential oil aromatherapy is a very complicated one as the use of the smoke has a very specific reason. A cleansing smoke bath will purify the body, aura and energy in a space. In the US we associate smoke cleansing with Native American tribes. As well in ancient Greece smoke cleansing formed part of the rituals to contact the dead, following long periods of fasting and silence. Many African cultures also use smudging on a daily basis. Ancient Celtic druids used sage and oak moss for burning and medicinal purposes. The smoke carries energy, both positive energies that we desire for a space, and carrying negative energies and vibrations out of a space. The idea of burning has to do with the element of fire which is the most purifying of all elements. The more you clear and balance your energy fields, the more attractive it becomes too negative ions due to the polarity of the different energies.

The theoretical direction of the electrical field flow is considered to be from positive to negative by convention, opposite to the flow of electrons. EMF is the flow of electrons, and low frequency EMFs are those that come from human-made electrical machines. These low frequencies cause an energy disruption in our energy fields because it is the natural order of energy. Aromatherapy, smoke cleansing, sound therapy, energy work and anything that helps to increase your higher vibrations will help with keeping us aligned. However they are not something that will keep the EMFs from doing what they do, and so it's a constant battle of balance. Over the last 30 years the concern that daily exposure to extremely low-frequency magnetic fields, considered to be 1 to 300 Hz, might be harmful to human health. Subtle aromatherapy is a great support tool, and so we shall continue to learn more.

The truth that we can heal, we must learn again. Medicine is in our hearts and also in the heart of that which we call the Universe.

Nikola Tesla stated that, "The truth that we can heal, we must learn again. Medicine is in our hearts and also in the heart of that which we call the Universe." With that thought, we are given a higher purpose. E=mc2 which proved that mass and energy are interchangeable, and that time and space are not absolute. If you can slow down the alpha and beta waves of your brain you can create an electromagnetic release from all time, space and dimensions.

Electrophysiological studies using aroma with EKGs have revealed that various aromas affect spontaneous brain activities and cognitive functions. Our thoughts, emotions and behavior are the reflection of neuronal activity within the brain. So what else is possible when you add aromatherapy into your practice?

10

EMOTIONAL SUPPORT

If we are filled with energy centers, pathways and receptors, then it makes sense that there could be a connection between emotions and energy. When you have an emotional response you are actually reacting to incoming smells, sounds, movement and other inputs of awareness. Your amygdala doesn't care if it sees a real threat, or just a perceived threat. The reaction will be the same.

Before you actually even see danger visually, your amygdala and hypothalamus are already in action. The amygdala sprints off a message to the hypothalamus to let everyone in the nervous system know that we need the energy right now to flee, or fight. However, we have a neural pathway and mechanism that can change that. This input from the heart to the brain can inhibit or facilitate our brain's electrical activity. In 1974, French researchers stimulated the vagus nerve which carries many of the signals from the heart to the brain in cats and found that the brain's electrical response was reduced to about half its normal rate. Deep breathing exercises stimulate our vagus nerve. Add that to the knowledge that the practice of breathing can calm our brain.

A study in 2016 found the neural circuit in the brainstem that they are now calling the brain's "breathing pacemaker". The circuit can influence emotional states just by altering our breathing rhythm. Teaching mindful awareness starts with biohacking your flee or fight response from the amygdala and instead moving the response to the prefrontal cortex to be conscious in our reaction. Our prefrontal cortex is a big deal. It's very large because it's there to help us solve, plan and think carefully. The trick for using that big resource for our body is that the amygdala has to be calm in order to send the information on. If we introduce the inhaled essential oil to be absorbed by olfactory system into the central nervous system it can modulate our neuronal excitability, or control the neurotransmitter releasing process, which we know due to several essential oil studies on Bergamot, True Lavender and Juniper essential oils.

There are so many pathways that can take information to the amygdala. From the vagus nerve, facial input, taste input, or area postrema which monitors blood, food poisoning, motion sickness and vomiting... all of these different inputs within the medulla oblongata move information into what are called the nucleus of tractus solitarius or NTS. The NTS also receives input from heart, lungs, nerves, receptors, respiratory tracts and our face. Some of this information can then go directly to the amygdala, but sometimes it has to go through many of subcortical layers out of the medulla oblongata. The information may end up as fear or anxiety in the thalamus, or it may end up in the hypothalamus. However only olfactory input goes directly to the amygdala and creates an emotional perception. This is the brilliance of essential oils and aromatherapy.

This heart-brain sends more information to your regular brain, than your regular brain sends to the heart. The heart is in charge. Three 10-

year studies found that emotional stress is more predictive of death from cancer or cardiovascular disease than from smoking.

So how does our heart communicate with the brain? There are several different ways including nerve impulses, hormones and transmitters, through pressure waves and electromagnetic field interactions. Through the research in this field we know that when we are near another being our cardiorespiratory and brainwave patterns sync up. Our two hearts beat as one, as they say. Through BioAcoustic research our heart and brain will synchronize to the right beat frequency.

We have confirmed the existence of a wide range of communication means used by plants, including quantum-assisted magnetic and/or acoustic sensing and signaling. Measured sound emissions by plants as well as differential germination rates, growth rates and behavioral modifications in response to sound are well documented, and over 2000 plants species have evolved buzz pollination in which they release pollen from anthers only when vibrated at a certain frequency created exclusively by bee flight muscles. Since plant roots respond only to sound waves at frequencies that match waves emitted by the plants themselves, we must hypothesis that this bioacoustic connection could hold the key to the energetic value of using essential oils.

Plants emit audio acoustic emissions between 10–240 Hz and essential oils range in frequency from 52 up to 580 MHz.

A radiologist from Stockholm, Bjorn Nordenstrom, wrote the book Biologically Closed Circuits. He discovered in the 1980's that by putting an electrode inside a tumor and running a milliamp Direct

Current through the electrode, he could dissolve the cancer tumor and stops its growth. He also found electropositive and electronegative energy fields in the human body.

Tainio Technology in Cheney, Washington developed new equipment to measure the bio frequency of humans and foods. It has been used to determine the relationship between frequency and disease while measuring their frequencies. The human body frequency when it lowers to below 58 Hz, you will see that the immune system is compromised in some manner. The idea is that this measurable frequency is this body that we live in. Over this last year I started using Quantum Biofeedback in my own practice, and was honestly surprised at how accurate this was at sensing what was going on in my body via my energetic field. I was turned on to this by a Holistic Psychiatrist and am grateful that there are many more open minds in today's world than there used to be. Perhaps it is that so many people are awakening.

Each of our organs is in tune to a specific frequency, and so using aromatherapy as a vibrational tuner is something that is measurable as an important role in the therapeutic activity. You do not need to be a doctor to understand the balance of an energetic being, nor are you healing the body when you use an essential oil with the intention of balance. A study showed that after massage with a carrier oil that had diluted lavender essential oils in it, the main ingredients of linalool and linalyl acetate were detected in the blood within five minutes and peaked at 20 minutes; by 90 minutes, they were mostly eliminated. Another experiment confirmed immediate blood pressure lowering effects within 10 minutes of essential oil inhalation. It also showed the presence of the ingredients of essential oil in blood within five minutes after inhalation along with a reduction in stress reaction.

Oil frequencies are documented in these books: The Essential Oil Desk Reference, published by Essential Science Publishing 2001; and Reference Guide for Essential Oils, by Connie and Alan Higley, Revised edition 2001.

Robyn Openshaw, the author of the book "Vibe" says, "*Since oils are the highest energetic part of plants, it's a concentration in high vibrational frequency and may be a useful part of your goal to improve your grounding and your high, consistent, steady frequency.*"

An essential oil like lavender with so much research associated with it, and as such can be seen as one of the top oils people feel connected to. Lavender has a frequency of 118 MHz. True lavender essential oil offers a soothing aroma which makes it an appropriate frequency for a nervous feeling and emotions of anxiety. This favorite oil calms my mind, and releases mental exhaustion. Lavender essential oil is one of the go to oils for meditation, mediumship and raising our spiritual connections.

Psychologists from Wesleyan University ran a sleep study on thirty one individuals. They were asked to inhale lavender essential oil before going to bed and then simply inhale distilled water the following night. The scientists monitored their sleep patterns using brain scans. What they found was that the individuals when inhaling the lavender slept more soundly and reported feeling more energetic the next morning.

So if we go back to research on Lavender and the nervous system, scientists believe lavender stimulates the activity of brain cells in the amygdala similar to the way some sedative medications work. The rate of overdose deaths from anti-anxiety drugs increased fourfold from 1996 to 2013. More than one in five American adults took medications for psychiatric disorders such as anxiety and depression in 2010. In a study published in the journal Phytomedicine, lavender oil was shown to be just as effective as the pharmaceutical drug Ativan. As well it showed no sedative effects, which is a common side effect, and it had no potential for drug abuse or dependence. The more we learn about our beings, the more we understand the benefits of essential oils.

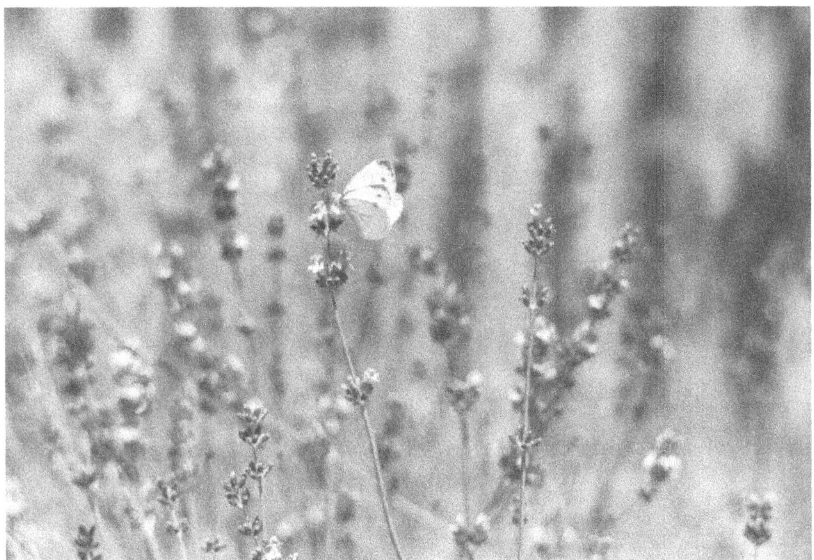

We are made of peptides. These peptides are really just short little pieces of proteins. There are no dangerous elements in peptides. They are made of amino acids, and these are made of the same elements that make up human beings. The pattern of the "beads on the string" is what makes peptides bioactive. While essential oils are much smaller than peptides, when you apply an undiluted essential oil on your skin organic compounds within the essential oil can combine with peptides in the skin to form a new molecule, called a peptide-hapten complex.

A hapten is a minute molecule that can elicit an immune response only when attached to a large carrier such as a protein. Developing a contact allergy to an essential oil is mainly due to the exposure frequency and sensitizing capacity of the sensitizing chemical, the hapten, through neat skin application. This is what happens when undiluted oils create a response in the skin, and this is where a misconception that you cannot become allergic to an essential oil happens. Please do not slather yourself with undiluted essential oils thinking that as a vibrational being you can handle it. This just isn't the case. If you consider that there are so many synthetic lavender oils being sold on the market today, and look at the research, this is the biggest risk we have with skin care products and fragrances being added to them. This is similarly the consideration with oral use of essential oils.

A pro-hapten is not chemically reactive and cannot form a covalent bond with a peptide. To become chemically reactive, they must first be converted into a hapten by being metabolized into a compound that is chemically reactive. Pro-haptens are found in pharmacological interactions of drugs with immune receptors. It is important to distinguish between peptide-haptens and prohaptens. The only risk in research at this time in regards to essential oils and pro-haptens are through impurities or oxidation products in the synthetic items. Purity matters so much, for so many reasons. Frequency, safety, therapeutic abilities come from nature.

A great place to start your practice is to use aromatherapy with the idea of balancing the energy bodies. The olfactory system was created as such an aligned mechanism for using essential oils safely. Start looking at frequencies, chakras and emotions as another guide when choosing an essential oil that will support the body, and the heart-brain connection.

11

OIL IDENTIFICATION

Now we come to the part of just what each essential oil is capable of, and what energies you can use them for. This will be where you come back again and again to reference oils as you first start to work with oils in your daily routine.

NOTE: With all internal usage information, it is up to you to work with your Certified Aromatherapist to be assured of purity, and your Pharmacist to make sure there will not be any interactions with your medications or supplementation.

1)ATLAS CEDARWOOD

Cedrus atlantica

One of the most majestic oils, this oil found its way into my routine when my husband was suffering with the tension associated with a spasming shoulder. The grounding abilities of this oil added to a personal blend offered him a calming and soothing feeling for both body and mind.

My favorite oil, produced mostly from Moroccan wood, is steam distilled with the main Sesquiterpene constituents of Beta, Alpha and Gamma Himachalene, however it also has Sesquiterpene ketones and should not be used with those that are sensitive to these oils. It is also not to be used in pregnant women or babies due to the neurotoxic and abortive properties.

Atlas cedarwood is a conifer. A Conifer is a tree that bears cones and evergreen needlelike or scale like leaves. This tree is usually seen throughout the Middle East and the Himalayas, and has acclimated to Europe.

Atlas Cedarwood should only be used aromatically, diluted topically, however is never used internally. It is often used in beauty products like massage oils, skin care and hair care due to the aromatic compounds. It is a base note for use for any grounding blends, and a wonderful oil to use with root chakra energy work.

2) BALSAM FIR
Abies balsamea

This is such an uplifting fragrance, and as such, Balsam Fir is one that I love to use during the winter season for its supportive properties. This comes from its main terpene properties of a-pinene and b-pinene, as well as its Delta-3-Carene. These all are bicyclic monoterpene. These terpenes are something we tend to seek out when we are looking for that respiratory support or a little extra focus and memory retention.

Delta-3 Carene is known to support those seeking anti-inflammatory support. This terpene is found in cannabis and pine oils as well. In 2008 a study looked at Delta-3 Carene and suggests that this terpene speeds up the healing of bones, especially for those that suffer from malnourishment. Not surprising, it also offers intestinal support.

Distilled from needles and leaves, this oil was often used in sacred rituals, and is one I often use in energy work. As a major support for releasing obstacles in the sacral and heart chakras, this oil is balancing to the subtle body energies. Use it to not only increase a joyful mood, but dilute topically to help increase the movement within the body. Diffuse it when sitting in front of your light therapy in those long, dark winter months. Balsam Fir can be used as an aromatherapy oil, diluted for topical use, or add a drop into your warm tea or a veggie capsule for internal support. Always ask seek advice from your Certified Aromatherapist and Pharmacist to discuss interactions before starting any essential oil internal use.

3) BERGAMOT
Citrus bergamia
Citrus Bergamot is a highly researched oil. It has been used in clinical experiments against lice and other parasites, to reduce anxiety during radiation treatments, and so much more. As a citrus oil it is cold pressed from the peel, and one of the most versatile citrus oils, and generally from Italy. However, it's photosensitizing properties means that you should avoid the sun if you are using it on your skin for several hours.

Bergamot is mostly a monoterpene, which is limonene. Limonene is a powerful component and can be found in more than just the citrus oils. You can find limonene in fir needles, cannabis, palo santo and Frankincense carterii. Using this oil during meditation can effectively work with the root chakra, brow chakra, crown chakra and those upper aura chakras that connect directly into the divine energy. This protective oil is supportive of the physical body as a Monoterpene, and I love blending high limonene oils like Bergamot and Frankincense carterii for general support of head discomfort.

You will often find Bergamot being used in deodorants as it is a natural for eliminating odors. Try using this oil before walking on stage to perform; speaking in public or anytime you feel the need for a boost in confidence. Bergamot can be use aromatically, diluted well as it is strong oil for topical use, or you can add a drop in a veggie capsule to support appetite regulation, and minimize digestive disturbances.

4) BLACK PEPPER

Piper nigrum

How many times have you seen the use of adding pepper to help the bioavailability of a supplement? From Brazil, Malaysia, Madagascar and especially India the black pepper plants grow as a vine several feet tall. Used for both culinary and medicinal purposes, these peppercorns have been used by Indian monks for thousands of years to support their daily endurance.

From the vine this fruit gives black, white and red or pink peppercorns depending on the season and how they plant is grown. A stimulating and warm oil, it is often used in cooking to give a spicy nudge to a dish. It offers deep emotional balance, and helps release stuck cellular energies that are creating rigid patterns in your life. Using this in connection with both the root chakra and the third eye chakra can give you a deep connection to both Earth and spirit.

This oil has high Sesquiterpene and Monoterpene properties. ß-caryophyllene, its Sesquiterpene component, is known as a dietary cannabinoid. When looking at the most distinct cannabinoids on the market today, this is the compound that plays the role of reducing those anxious feelings as it has the ability to bind to our CB2 receptors. I love that this oil has decent amounts of a-pinene properties. A-pinene has been used in synergy with cannabinoids in MRSA experiments as they have a high synergistic effect. Add in the benefits of high monoterpene limonene and you have one of the best oils to have in your home arsenal.

Black pepper essential oil can be diluted well for use topically to help support digestion, promote relief to sore muscles or even support seasonal respiratory functions. It can be used aromatically for stimulation and normal respiratory support, as well as added to any dish after cooking for a savory flavor to your meal.

5) BLUE TANSY

Tanacetum annum

Blue tansy is actually blue, and is steam distilled from the flower and stems of the plant that originated in the Mediterranean, although it is a plant native to various parts of Europe. As an oil with camphor, which is a ketone, this oil should not be used for those with sensitivities to neurotoxic oils. This includes those with seizures, even though it is low in thujones. Also because of this reason it is not recommended to be used during pregnancy, or with those with endocrine dysfunction. This oil is not recommended for use with young children.

The Sesquiterpene chamazulene (pronounced sha-ma-za-lean) is restorative and often used in skin care as an herbal remedy additive. It is this property that creates the blue in the chamomile flower. Blue is the color of healers, and there seems to be a reason why Blue Tansy is such a useful oil for unblocking energies. Like drinking a glass of fine wine, this oil's aroma can relax you and even open up that throat chakra to allow you speak your truth. It opens up natural instincts through the first chakra, and connects us with an awareness of higher energies. This makes the blue tansy a wonderful oil for anyone trying to increase their intuitive nature, or when doing energy work or intuitive readings.

Blue tansy is mostly monoterpenes, including b-pinene and sabinene, which gives the oil the benefits to the skin to soothe everything from insect bites to sore muscles and is very supportive to respiratory functions. I think of Blue Tansy as an alternative to Helichrysum italicum for the skin. Blue Tansy can be used aromatically and topically and for adults can be used neat if desired. This oil should not be used internally.

6) CINNAMON

Cinnamomum verum

Cinnamomum verum comes from the Ceylon cinnamon bark grown in Sri Lanka, where it is extracted by steam distillation. When looking at cinnamon Ceylon is called true cinnamon and is considered very healthy, whereas cassia can be harmful in large amounts. Most cinnamon that you purchase in the United States is cassia.

My daughter calls this a very spicy oil, although it has a sweet component. This oil is mostly an aldehyde, which means it will irritate the skin. When used in clinical experimentation, it was found to reduce food intake, improve lipid parameters and lower blood glucose in diabetes-induced rats. It also contains smaller amounts of a Terpenic Ester and a Monoterpene, ß-phellandrene

Cinnamon is a very comforting aroma, and can help transform your belief system, especially when used in conjunction with energy work.

I use this oil when I am working with those clients dealing with limitations in their choices in regards to money, relationships, anger and feelings of frustration. It is such an empowering when working with the solar plexus to spark your own personal fire. As well many healers associate cinnamon as an energetic oil that can be used to ground the root chakra, and makes it a good choice to purify a space before or use at the end of the session to ground and cleanse.

Great oil to use for cleansing anything physical when you find a need. I love to use it on my counters as it has been tested extensively to be highly effective at controlling mold growth. This oil can be used aromatically for these purifying properties, highly diluted if you truly desire to use it topically to increase your energies, or one drop in warm tea or added at the end of cooking a dish to enhance flavor.

7) CITRONELLA

Cymbopogon winterianus

Cymbopogon winterianus, which is the Java type of Citronella, is a wonderful, complex yet lemony essential oil. This essential oil is highly Monoterpene aldehyde with the citronella, Monoterpene alcohol with both citronellol and geraniol, but with small amounts of the Monoterpene limonene and the terpene ester geranyl acetate.

Citronella is steam distilled from the grassy leaves and grown in Indonesia. The Citronella winterianus is the Java type which is darker in color than the sweeter Ceylon type, Citronella nardus. Just as you would use a citronella candle, this oil can be diluted and applied to your skin when you are going to be outdoors, however it is simply soothing on muscles and joints after you get done with you hike. I love using this oil as well to relieve tension, and as an uplifting and protective oil.

We work on our connections and our creations in our second chakra, and love, protection, happy thoughts in our fourth chakra. So it isn't any wonder that this oil is a wonderful fit for energy work in these areas. It can be used as a middle note, or even a top note. Make sure to dilute your Citronella since those aldehydes can be irritating on the skin when applied neat. Often this oil is added in a toner for its cleansing properties.

You can diffuse this oil to cleanse and purify your space before any energy work or based on the season, but you can also take a drop or two in a veggie capsule to support antioxidant function and the functions of the immune system. Such a vibrant oil, and one I love to have around.

8) CLARY SAGE
Salvia sclarea

One of the first times I shared Salvia sclarea was with a mom friend. She had two wildly active boys and was suffering with monthly female discomfort. I handed her the bottle and said, "I will watch the boys for a minute. Go into the bathroom and rub some of that on your lower abdomen (diluted of course)." She came back smiling, relaxed, and realized that this plant was like a miracle worker.

This is an oil that has been used since before the Middle Ages, and was once thought to reinforce your eyesight. The origin of the name, clear eye or Clary Sage, stems from the Latin word "clarus", or clear. It is very transformative when used aromatically with work using the third eye chakra for insight, to gain perspective or reflect inward to see truth and expand your possibilities.

Clary Sage comes from the flowering tops of the plant, and is steam distilled. Offers the Monoterpene alcohol linalool, it carries similarities to True Lavender as a third eye opener. Also very high in Esters, including linalyl acetate, which gives us those calming mood and emotional support, as well has supporting to our hormone functions. Clary sage also stimulates your root chakra, your sacral chakra and the solar plexus chakra. One of the most aligning aromas to the entire subtle body, it is a very useful oil to the energy worker's arsenal.

Clary Sage has a wonderful bicyclic Sesquiterpene, cadinene, which is surprisingly used in cigarettes and alcoholic beverages as a favorite industry flavoring. This compound can be found in similar amounts in Ylang Ylang II or Ylang Ylang III, Atlas Cedarwood, Juniper Berry and Melissa. Often this compound is discussed in broad strokes to refer to any Sesquiterpene with the cadalane carbon skeleton, although it is actually a subclass of that compound. This not so secret information is used in the distillation industry as the compound that completes the flavor of the oil. Interesting that in Chinese Traditional Medicine Clary Sage is known for strengthening and completing the circulation of our Ki. Remember that Ki is the universal life force energy that flows through each and every one of us, everything, and beyond.

Often Clary Sage essential oil is adulterated, and so knowing the purity of this oil is vital to its efficacy and safety. With a pure, and toxin-free product you can use this oil in the safe bath protocols I referred to in earlier chapters, and soak to soothe those sore muscles after a workout, due to common menstrual cycle symptoms or just because it feels good. However because of the way this oil works with the menstrual cycle, it should be avoided in pregnant women, women who are nursing, children and those dealing with cancer, inflammation of the breast tissues. When diluted well it can be used topically, which I see most often in my Aromatherapy practice, or aromatically

9) CLOVE

Syzygium aromaticum

Syzygium aromaticum is a very widely known essential oil, and highly favored as both a cooking spice, and for holistic benefits. Steam distilled generally from Indonesian clove buds; this botanical has been studied for its anti-inflammatory properties, cellular protection, and soothing nature to respiratory and intestinal function. Ask an aroma dealer, and they are likely to say they use it topically for oral support to reduce pain and tenderness due to its numbing properties.

The trees that provide the flowering clove buds often stay productive for 150 years. One of the main "spicy" oils, it is considered to be a warming oil energetically and physically. No matter if you need to ground out, soothe emotions, or open up your perspective; clove is a wonderful aroma to diffuse for these reasons.

Clove oil is made up mostly of eugenol, with smaller amounts of eugenol acetate. It is balanced by the small amounts of Sesquiterpenes, which provide a grounded metal clarity as well as increases the cleansing and energetic circulation of Ki. If you are struggling to get over emotional pain in your journey, you may want to use some Clove oil aromatically to help reduce the emotional pull long enough to do the work you are called to.

It is important to note that Phenols are very irritating and require high levels of dilution. Even with the highly spicy nature this oil is sought out for protection from environmental, oxidizing and cellular threats, as has been used as far back as 200 BC in China. With pure oils, you may use Clove internally as well in small amounts at the end of cooking a dish you wish to season, or in a veggie capsule followed by an oil chaser. When I refer to an oil chaser it is just a tbsp. or internally applicable oil that will help coat and dilute Clove in the digestive tract.

10) COPAIBA

Copaifera langsdorffii

Copaifera langsdorffii has to be one of my top five essential oils of all time. It is just recently starting to gain attention for its ability to connect to the CBD-2 receptors. When we think of CBD, we first think of steam distilled or carbon dioxide distilled hemp seed oil. Beta-caryophyllene is a Sesquiterpene that connects to most notably that CB2 human receptor that works with the brain, spine, gut, and reproductive systems. When looking at hemp based CBD oil companies are only recently looking for what they call the Entourage Effect. This is a broad spectrum approach where the oil is over 80% wide spectrum terpenes and just 20% cannabinoids.

Cannabinoids activate human receptors that also work with the tonsils, spleen, blood cells, bones, muscles, tissues, endocrine system, skin, digestive tract, lungs, kidneys and even the brain and nervous system. The difference between the Beta-Caryophyllene cannabinoid and the THC cannabinoid, which is similar to anandamide, named after the Sanskrit term "Ananda," which translates to "peace", is obviously is how it impacts the brain through the CB1 receptors. You will not get high off of Copaiba essential oils because it does not impact that CB1 receptor.

So ß-caryophyllene is a terpene, and it is known as that first dietary cannabinoid. When you look at the HS-GS testing on your high quality THC-free CBD oil it generally has about a 0.2% total terpene weight, which most of that being isopulegol and menthol, and a minute amount ß-caryophyllene. When testing a Copaiba essential oil it can be as much as 60% ß-caryophyllene. CBD oils are generally diluted with carrier oils such as hemp seed or coconut oil, or purified water. This is why the oil that arrives at your home, or that you pick up at the local store contains such a low volume of this essential terpene.

Copaifera langsdorffii is tapped like maple syrup from the Balsam of the Rashed or Salem tree in South America where they grow up to 100 feet tall in the Amazonian rainforest. Working with a distributor that works hand in hand with the country to protect the rainforest is essential when using Copaiba. In a 2012 BMC Complementary and Alternative Medicine journal there was an article that showed that C. langsdorffii extract significantly reduced the extent of DNA damage and ACF, which are clusters of abnormal tube-like glands in the lining of the colon and rectum, when used with rats that had been induced with preneoplastic lesions. It showed up as having a protective effect, and I find that Copaiba essential oil offers that same protective and uplifting energy to the user's subtle body. It also promotes normal intestinal and respiratory function, and soothes and tightens skin.

Aromatically this oil is very grounding and balancing. When used in energy work it can open up a closed off client with generational walls built up, and is a perfect oil to send home to use during their meditation practice. It helps us see how we connect genetically, but separate our generational ties. This is such a beneficial aroma to use with the root, sacral and solar plexus imbalances. Besides aromatic use, this oil can also be used topically diluted, and internally when using a pure essential oil product.

11) CORIANDER

Coriandrum sativum

When people think of Coriandrum sativum, or Coriander seed oil, they often just think, weird. Coriander is a Mediterranean plant which is part of the parsley family. This oil is the steam distilled oil from the seeds, rather than from the leaf of the plant.

Coriandrum sativum is historically linked to the Ayurveda practice and is said to have be used over 7,000 years ago. If you think of this as an Ayurvedic oil, Coriander balances all three doshas. The doshas are Vata, Kapha and Pitta and are connected to the five elements of nature. You can use Coriander seed oil when it is transparently tested internally or at the end of cooking an Asian or Indian dish for a lovely sweet aroma, and a warm spicy kick.

Coriander seed oil will help you clear obstacles and help circulate that energy moving from the root chakra up through your crown chakra and beyond. As an energy worker I love adding this into a blend to use in a session for someone that struggles with receiving. Since it is mostly Monoterpene linalool, consider this the warner top and middle note sibling to True Lavender. Linalool has two stereoisomers that are licareol which is also called R-linalool, and coriandrol is called S-linalool.

Coriander seed oil is high a high Monoterpene, mostly the linalool we just discussed. As a Monoterpene you will use this oil for cleansing and stimulating needs. A stimulating oil helps move our Ki, and helps remove excessive negative emotions. Linalool is a protective compound, and protects cells in our nervous system as multiple studies have demonstrated that it can prevent disturbed nerve cell activity in the brain. When you are working in a high EMF area, diffusing linalool-rich oils can be supportive as these frequencies can damage the structure and function of the nervous system.

Coriandrum sativum also has a-pinene and camphor in its properties. Camphor is a ketone and so it should not be used with those sensitive to Monoterpene ketones including those that are pregnant, children and those that may have seizures.

You can also use Coriander seed oil diluted well topically to promote restoration in the body when you have overdone it. It also can be diffused to help with occasional feelings of nausea. As a healthy product it can be used internally when needed. My favorite way to use Coriander is to add in citrus and aromatically engage your space for a mood boost, cleansing, and protective support.

12) CYPRESS

Cupressus sempervirens

I moved back to Utah before having my daughter, and the first person I met at the model home office from the neighborhood ended up being my neighbor. Living right across the street, our daughters became and are still amazing friends, as are we. This big hearted warrior first introduced me to essential oils, and Cupressus sempervirens was the first oil that I knew intuitively she needed. Cypress oil helps with normal circulation, as you have guessed by now moving our energy force opens up a sense of security and stability. Energy often gets by our thoughts. Many cultures believe that swelling is a signal of this trapped energy.

Cupressus sempervirens, grown in Spain, is distilled from the twigs and shrubbery of the cypress tree. This rich oil has a delightfully piney scent that I love to diffuse during the holiday season. High in the Monoterpenes a-pinene and delta-3-carene

13) EUCALYPTUS GLOBULUS

Eucalyptus globulus

An overused oil in the eucalyptus family, Eucalyptus globulus is what you think of when you think of vapor rubs as the oil that supports healthy respiratory function. It has a fresh scent, but isn't for use in children, especially those under age ten. A steam distilled oil from the leaves of the evergreen eucalyptus tree, it is a native Australian oil, which has moved globally in the past several centuries.

This oil is mostly a Terpene Oxide, and contains a high percentage of eucalyptol. It also has a-pinene and limonene Monoterpenes as lessor chemical components. Used in purification, this oil still has a calming effect on both mind and body. This essential oil can be heavily diluted to be added to a muscle blend to relieve sore muscles after exercise.

This oil is most often thought of for respiratory support, and so it's not surprising that this oil works well for the Heart Chakra. Also this oil can open up your creator energy in the Sacral Chakra and combined can work magic with relationship obstacles that have blocked the connection of these two areas. As well, whenever you see oils that are meant to open us up, you are working with what I call a clarity oil. It will offer you expansion and a new perspective if you are seeking one.

14) FRANKINCENSE FREREANA

Boswellia frereana

As one of the varieties of Frankincense that is used across the board, this oil has a fruitier undertone than others you come across. Extracted from resin, and one of the most sacred essential oils, this oil offers you everything from protection to a release of emotions. If we consider the way that the oil comes to be, like the hearty wild blueberries, the resin of the Frankincense tree hardens into tears, or the blood of the tree. This energy carries with it into the oil an energy that is high in frequency for all emotional needs.

If you have ever seen what happens when a cell is exposed to a molecule of Frankincense it is incredible. The cell changes in color and become active in many ways due to the more than two hundred molecular compounds within this oil. Generally this oil is wild harvested from Somalia, and grows across the mountains alongside livestock. This highly sought after aroma was used by the Christian churches in the Middle Ages, for purification.

This oil is high in Monoterpenes, including the Monoterpene a-thujene and d-sabinene. The higher the amounts of a-thujene, the more likely the resin came from a female tree. This chemical is where soothing, reduction in inflammation and protection against harmful germs and bacteria comes from. A bicyclic monoterpene, d-sabinene, is where the oil get the properties for antibacterial, anti-fungal and other such benefits like stimulation of saliva, and opening up the pores.

Boswellia frereana will balance your chakras from root to crown, and can be used to help focus in for those a-type meditators. It offers a way to cleanse your subtle energy body, and connect in a calm manner for intuitive work. Yet this oil is very protective and purifying for the empathic and open intuitive worker.

15) FRANKINCENSE CARTERII

Boswellia carterii

A favorite oil, probably one of my first favorite oils. One I offer with a free diffuser through my partnership. A wonderful top note that everyone seems to love, as it works quickly with the limbic system to work on emotions, behavior, creativity and can spark long term memory. It is the lightest aromatic Frankincense, and as with all is similar to what I just shared above in being protective, grounding and able to purify a space.

Highly monoterpene, with lots of a-pinene, it penetrates the tissues quickly, and is a long lasting essential oil. Frankincense does everything from grounding to connecting to the pure source energy. I love to use it for meditation and when I need a little extra mental support. It's a great oil to add to an aroma bracelet or necklace to use to relieve the anxiety that comes on in crowds or new situations. All Frankincense oils offer us a way to cleanse our subtle energy body, and connect in a calm manner for intuitive work. Yet this oil is very protective and purifying for the empathic and open intuitive worker.

16) EUCALYPTUS RADIATA

Eucalyptus radiata

When working with those looking to support their respiratory system, this is my favorite oil to select and share. Eucalyptus radiata is mostly Oxides, with undertones of high amounts of Monoterpene, and very small amounts of Esters, Aldehydes and Sesquiterpenes. Distilled from Australian eucalyptus leaves, and is soothing although still needs to be diluted as a sensitive oil.

This oil has mostly eucalyptol, and due to the 1,8 cineole content, use caution with this oil.

Used in purification, this oil still has a calming effect on both mind and body. This oil can be heavily diluted to be added to a muscle blend to relieve sore muscles after exercise for many reasons, including the uplifting chakra benefits. Very connected to our Throat chakra, which is very yang energy connected to speaking your truth, this oil can be used to support gaining clarity, and energizing your subtle body. As well this version of eucalyptus promotes pure love. That is why when we balance our heart chakra we will sense less anxiety, less upper body issues, less fatigue and of course why this oil is so great for respiratory support.

17) GERANIUM

Pelargonium graveolens

A must oil for any woman's oil kit, this oil is steam distilled from the leaves and flowers of the geranium. This oil is a beautiful, floral aroma that will dominate a blend. It is about half Monoterpenols, with other Esters as its main components. This is my maca of essential oils, and very supportive for both women and men when it comes to supporting our hormone balance. It is regenerative in both body and spirit, and as such should be considered for those that are working through sorrow, low moods and energetic obstacles that are impeding the flow of Ki.

When we look at how this oil works within in the Sacral Chakra, it makes sense why every woman needs this oil in their routines. Pelargonium graveolens can boost energy; reduce lower body pains, and helps with digestive support. I shared with a family member that had major digestive issues, and was an immediate support tool in her herbal tea. It is being looked into with studies to see if this essential oil might have significant potential in developing new anti-inflammatory drugs, with lower side effects.

You can work with this oil when you are trying to work on creation, is uplifting and balancing. A wonderful oil to incorporate for couples energy work. Pelargonium graveolens gives you a protective layer of energy, and purifies a space after your intuitive work.

18) GERMAN CHAMOMILE

Matricaria recutita

This beautiful deep blue essential oil is a wonderful addition to your collection. This steam distilled flower is high in Sesquiterpenes and Oxides, and delivers topical and aroma support in so many ways that is often used in blends just to create possibilities of something more. However as much as I love what this oil offers, it is important to note that there are those with detoxification mutations that need to be aware of caution when using this oil. The enzyme we call CYP2D6 is a very important enzyme in the detoxification pathways. When you have this enzyme and you take a regular dose of a medication, your body works as it should work using the drug and clearing it out.

With this genetic mutation your body with active drugs your body can use a much lower dosage, and with drugs that the enzyme activates you may need more of the drug. So when you are taking a drug that requires activation by this enzyme, this can be a drug interaction. Imagine if you are taking a sleeping medication that requires a higher does, and Matricaria recutita instead makes you overly sleepy? If you are taking a antiplatelet or anticoagulant medication what if Matricaria recutita increases the effect and makes you more susceptible to bruising and bleeding? It can even cause some problems with anesthesia, and should not be used before surgery. Here is another case where knowing your genetic makeup can be helpful in guiding your essential oil selection,

When there are no interactions to worry about, this European originated oil offers support when traveling for irritable stomachs, anxious feelings and restless energy. Its anti-inflammatory properties make it wonderful for muscles, monthly pains, promoting respiratory support and it's not surprising as this oil works highly in the Heart and Throat Chakras. How often do you feel that you are floating in the wind, alone, while seeking out acceptance and love? This oil will offer an opportunity to clear the empty, isolating emotions and create a connection to self-love. Proper dilution is essential, but this oil can be used for an aroma blend or before any activity where you desire a deeper connection.

Use this oil when you are doing grounding exercises or meditation, and to offer a protective barrier for an open empathic that has not yet learned how to properly shield their emotional center. As the sensitive oil you can add it to an aroma charm and use as needed throughout the day. Can be diffused, applied in a topical diluted carrier solution or use a drop internally when working with a physician or skilled Aromatherapist using the precautionary rules for those without genetic knowledge, but with detoxification blockages.

19) GINGER

Zingiber officinale

I use ginger root on a daily basis, as a nutrient support. Zingiber officinale is one essential oil that can be used in many of the ways that we traditionally use ginger root and ginger spices. The underground stem of the plant is steam distilled, and it's important to remember that when thinking about the energetic connection to this oil. This plant shoots out its stems below the surface sending out lateral shoots and additional roots and intervals. When this plant senses that it needs new shoots to grow upwards, it just allows it and then it develops horizontal buds to create. Of course that means that Zingiber officinale works from the Root Chakra upwards, and creates balance in the energetic fields of the body.

I love using Ginger essential oil when working with individuals that come from unconnected family spaces. Touching on the most basic of survival needs, this oil allows the energy body to know that it is safe, and connected to all of us, especially source. This oil creates deeper relationships, harbors unconditional love, and gives back the power to the energy body. Speaking your truth is a side effect of using Zingiber officinale.

Because this oil has such strong roots, it is a very powerful oil. This is why I prefer to use organic ginger root powder in my morning tea rather than ginger essential oil. Although it can be used highly diluted internally and topically, I find that this oil shines when used aromatically instead. Some oils are designed by nature to be more fluid, and this is one of them. Add a few drops to your diffuse and breathe in the particles of rejuvenation, and release the emotions that are depleting your Auric Field.

Understanding that this oil contains high Sesquiterpenes and Monoterpenes means it can be used in both as a Middle Note or a Base Note, which opens more possibilities when designing blends for your clients. Although a warm energetic oil, you may use this oil in any month, even if it isn't cold outside.

20) GRAPEFRUIT
Citrus × paradise
When you think of grapefruit you either get joyous, or crinkle your

nose thinking about how awful it was when you were six. However this cold-pressed citrus oil is something that as a nose crinkler I rather enjoy. Although a phototoxic oil, this oil is quite uplifting and creates and awakening in your energy field. It purifies, cleanses and brings helps clarify your inner knowing. It may interfere with some statins, and always refer to the safety information when newly working with essential oils.

Citrus × paradisi has been researched as an aroma supporter for releasing trapped emotions in your cells, or as we like to call it, being overweight. This is one of those items that I gleaned from my professor at Bastyr. The aroma of Citrus × paradisi relaxes our parasympathetic gastric nerve. This is important because our second brain communicates with the central nervous system through our parasympathetic nerve, using the vagus nerve. That butterfly feeling that you have, is your second brain at work. Don't be afraid of it, be aware of it and see what knowledge it is trying to share with you today.

Nootkatone has been called the most important grapefruit aroma, as it activates AMP-activated protein kinase . AMPK plays a key role as a master regulator of cellular energy homeostasis. When we have a decrease in cellular energy homeostasis, we create a corresponding modification in the bioelectrical field of our being. Parasites, genetic mutations, blood flow and so many other items can impact our homeostasis levels. Part of what AMPK does, it is tells the body to open the cells and grab ahold of some energy, which is sugar. While grapefruit essential oil does not burn fat, the only way to open our cells to burn that fat is to exercise to open and release energy or through insulin to activate storage of energy to use later. Having an assist to your functional and subtle body energy fields through and aromatic oil is quite a blessing.

As you can suspect, Citrus × paradisi is a beautiful Monoterpene. This aroma connects you to uplifting stored emotions and opens up the Heart Chakra to bring balance to your inner feelings of love. I recommend this oil to cleanse your space, cleanse your body, cleanse your Aura and create a possibility for releasing stored energy, and more. Use this oil topically, aromatically and internally when working with a physician or an Aromatherapist with a working knowledge of your wellness history.

21) HELICHRYSUM

Helichrysum italicum

One of my favorite stories of Helichrysum italicum is with a friend. She ran after her toddler on a hot summer day, barefoot, onto the hot asphalt. When we met up a few days later at a park playdate, her feet were a wreck. I gave her some Helichrysum italicum and told her that it was the only known essential oil that had clinical backing to rejuvenate cellular tissue. This oil gets use for facial serums, moisturizers, and body balms for exactly this reason. As her feet healed, she was intrigued by this little oil that did so much, so quickly.

I know that Helichrysum has been used internally, but I have never used it that way, nor recommended it to a customer. It never showed up in that manner in my internal knowing of an essential oil protocol. However, I do use it from time to time around my eyes, to keep people guessing about my external age.

Traditionally this is a Corsican steam distilled flower, but it is now being grown in many areas around the globe. Still highly priced, no matter which small batch or large organization you attain it from, this lovely yellow oil is mostly Esters, being highly neryl acetate. This is the component that was originally found in Neroli essential oil. This is the compound that offers the calming and soothing support to your skin. It can also offer high α-pinene compounds that we normally associate with coniferous trees. Some research has shown the ability of a-pinene to inhibit certain forms of cell death, and we are seeing a lot of new ideas for using a-pinene rich oils on the horizon.

Helichrysum is a high vibrational, highly energetic essential oil that will balance your entire energetic system. Regardless of if the imbalance is deeply rooted, or an intuitive need, using Helichrysum italicum in your practice will create an inner flow of energy that not many essential oils can offer. It calms, and restores, it protects and heals, and of course is transforms and creates through source energetic frequencies. As a quantum connector, this is an amazing aroma to diffuse during your biofeedback replay.

 As a costly oil, there are other alternatives that you can blend together to get many similar benefits to Helichrysum italicum, although if it calls to you I recommend you listen and gently place it on your oil shelf.

22) JUNIPER BERRY

Juniperus communis

Many years ago, in the heart of the aromatherapy revolution, hospitals in France would burn the sprigs of the juniper to purify and cleanse the air. Perhaps this comes from Psalms 120:4 where the juniper shrub was used to cleanse and purify and remove negative and false energy, through smoke. Juniper is a Native plant medicine, and used in cleansing rituals. Today many people use this oil to promote purification and respiratory support; however I love to use it for the energetic response for underlying stress.

Juniperus communis has very high levels of Monoterpenes and is mostly completed with Sesquiterpenes, and steam distilled from the berries and needles of the juniper shrubs/trees. It is mainly calming and grounding. When my husband was dealing with a shoulder injury and his doctor just didn't know what to offer, I blended several oils together and included Juniperus communis to help release the stress he was holding onto. I found that as he became stressed out about the pain and spasms, he would tense up. Aromatherapy offered an emotional support to let go of the fear, and lessened the tension. Grounding him in the protection of the Root Chakra gave a support for the physical body.

Juniper essential works with the Root Chakra, and the Solar Plexus Chakra to create some amazing benefits. In our Solar Plexus lives our spleen. The spleen chakra draws in the air prana for the rest of the body. When we are worried, anxious and overthinking, it create imbalance in the spleen chakra, which we often see as digestive distress. When our spleen and stomach are damaged or out of balance, it is believed that we leak our true Ki. Interestingly enough, when we have a leaky gut it creates a functional train wreck in the body and serious trouble with all of your energetic and physical systems. Juniperus communis promotes normal intestinal function, and rebalances the Solar Plexus.

You may diffuse, dilute and rub on your stomach, or add a drop into a favorite meal or veggie capsule to offer your Meridians the opportunity to clear out blockages and open up to flow.

23) LEMON

Citrus × limon

When you think about a most used oil, you think about Citrus × limon. Lemon essential oil is another phototoxic essential oil that is cold pressed from the citrus peel. Mostly Monoterpenes, including d-Limonene, this oil is a highly used oil for its cleansing properties. Lemon essential oil has been used for these cleansing properties for thousands of years. This uplifting essential oil is often used in homemade cleaners because it gives such a fresh scent to any area you use it, but that aroma does not last long. Citrus oils are highly evaporative.

Citrus × limon has been used in many clinical research studies. One study several years ago was to find out how well the aroma of this oil could help with morning sickness. The study found that this oil is effective in reducing nausea and vomiting for women that were pregnant. It has also been recommended by medical professionals for headaches and mental fatigue.

It also has been tested in lowering levels of corticosterone, which is a hormone secreted by the adrenal cortex. When looking into how this would work with anxiety, they found that lemon essential oil may possess anxiety-reducing and pain-relieving properties.

Studies looking into prenatal high corticosterone showed that high corticosterone levels in prenatally stressed rats predict persistent paradoxical sleep alterations, also known as known as REM sleep or dreaming sleep. This predisposed them to long-lasting disturbances that persist throughout adulthood. This included high anxiety, dysfunction of the hypothalamus-pituitary-adrenal axis, and abnormal circadian timing. They looked at the similar sleep disturbances in depressed patients and found a parallel due to hypercortisolemia and sleep alterations these patients can relate to stress-inducing events. So although lemon essential oil may not be the first oil you consider using for relaxation and quality sleep, it may be one that you should start to consider using.

A highly energetic essential oil for the Crown and Third Eye Chakras, Citrus × limon can help you when seeking clarity and inspiration. It also offers a subtle energy for creation connection your higher knowledge to our Sacral Chakra, breathing energy into a project or opening possibilities for a new experience.

Lemon essential oil can be used aromatically, topically when diluted and when staying covered from the sun, and internally when working with a medical professional or Certified Aromatherapist.

24) LEMONGRASS

Cymbopogon flexuosus

Lemongrass is the little essential oil that creates an exceptional ability to focus. A beautiful, earthy scent, this aroma is composed of high amounts of Aliphatic Aldehyde. This has a slightly different makeup than your normal Aldehyde, because it doesn't have an adjacency to an aromatic ring. This is great because it gives it a greater electrophilicity which means it is an electron lover. Since we are made of electrons and other atomic particles, this oil becomes a highly conductive aroma for the clairvoyant practitioner or energy worker.

This oil is grounding and uplifting, rooting us in balance while opening up our Third Eye Chakra and developing a balanced perspective on any situation.

Studies indicate that Lemongrass essential oil possesses various pharmacological activities such as anti-amoebic, antibacterial, antidiarrheal, antifilarial, antifungal and anti-inflammatory properties. Shown to be effective for controlling Candida albicans growth, it has gained significance due to the resistance acquired by pathogens toward a number of widely used drugs. When you inhale this lovely essential oil before a stressful event, it has even been shown to prevent anxious emotions.

My first inhalation of Cymbopogon flexuosus made me think of eating Fruit Loops when I was six or seven on a Saturday morning while watching cartoons. When I would wear this aroma to my daughter's cooperative program, almost every mom would say, "Wow, you smell so good!" This aroma will take you to a happy space, and open up your heart. A very powerful support tool for your Heart Chakra, I love to use this oil when energetically working with those that have self-love issues, or when I am rebalancing my own Heart Chakra after an especially active session. This aroma is supportive in breaking down obstacles to self-worth, and money beliefs and is one that most young adults could use in their regular aroma usage.

Just a small drop internally can promote healthy digestive function; it is more often used aromatically than topically. I still love blending it with carrier oils and wearing it, or adding it to my aroma necklace because it is one of my favorite aromas on the planet.

25) LIME

Citrus aurantifolia

Another fantastic citrus peel oil for uplifting energies and working with childhood implants, many people reach for this oil when creating blends. This oil is one of the most clinically tested oils I have seen.

One of the studies I really want people to know about is the use of Citrus aurantifolia aerosol for significantly reducing cravings for cigarettes, and for enhancing smoking reduction and cessation with people trying to quit smoking cigarettes. Since half a million people die from tobacco use and exposure to secondhand smoke, it is important to know that there are natural support tools to help you overcome this addiction.

Citrus aurantifolia also possesses important spasmolytic properties, which means it relieves spasm of smooth muscle. In animal testing this was tested on the small intestine, aorta and uterus. Its antimicrobial activity has also been tested on Gram-positive bacteria, Gram-negative bacteria and yeasts. The researchers found good antimicrobial activity, in particular on Gram-positive bacteria including Staphylococcus aureus, Bacillus subtilis and Staphylococcus epidermidis. This is mostly likely do the limonene, b-pinene and g-terpinene. This Monoterpene essential oil is phototoxic, and should not be applied if you are going to be out in the sunshine, so get your Vitamin D boost before using this essential oil topically.

Citrus aurantifolia can help when your creativity feels blocked, or you want to crawl back into bed and sleep. When your aura is dusty, this is the aroma for you. It will help you resist building fake relationships, as well as guide you to speak your truth. It offers you an opportunity to cleanse your emotional baggage, balancing out your Heart Chakra and Throat Chakra. You can even use this to release tension in both body and mind. Can be used diluted without sun exposure topically, in small amounts internally, or aromatically to renew and uplift your energy field.

26) MARJORAM

Origanum majorana

This is another often underutilized essential oil. In India this is considered a functional food or nutraceutical. I try to always remember that micronutrients facilitate body processes. As an essential oil, Origanum majorana comes from the flowering plant and its leaves, with high Monoterpenol properties.

Monoterpenols are very skin friendly essential oils, think of geraniol or linalol. Terpinen-4-ol offers very healing benefits when using this oil topically. As the most active constituent of Tea Tree essential oil, Marjoram also possesses high amounts of this chemical component. The benefits are in the calm that this provides as an essential oil, energetically. Soothing to the both body and mind, I generally recommend that your oil collection contain Origanum majorana.

This essential oil also contains Monoterpene Hydrocarbons and Oxygenated Monoterpenes as well as Phenolic compounds. When we think of Monoterpene Hydrocarbons we often go right to the citrus oils which are quickly oxidized. However, Frankincense and Black Pepper oil are also two other great Monoterpene Hydrocarbon essential oils. The high Oxygenated Monoterpene essential oils are being tested for their potential antifungal agents for ringworm in designing new formulations for topical treatments. Ringworm is a fungus that invades keratinized tissue, which is the epidermis of our skin.

We also have a band of keratinized tissue around our teeth in the mucous membrane, although keratinized epithelium covers the entire surface of our body, including our hair. When you think of the barrier to prevent infection, while controlling the loss of waste and water, the forefront of this process to maintain homeostasis is the highly keratinized epidermis which is the center of the ecology influencing your skin microbiome. Is it no wonder then that this aroma can be used for energetic protection?

Use this aroma when creating a protective energy, or in an emotionally supportive blend due to its ability to overcome rigid beliefs, emotional blockages, deeply rooted emotional imbalance, and repetitive thoughts. Of course use this aroma as a shield due to the vibrational connection to our physical body protective layer. This aroma has an ability to open up our memories to allow us to speak to their truth. When you are in fear, and lack the gumption to take a stand, use this essential oil to your benefit. Those that feel closed off in their Sacral Chakra should add this essential oil into a daily aroma blend for diffusing or use in a roller bottle, and continue to use until the subtle energy field has returned to an open and flowing energy.

Origanum majorana is most often used diluted for topical massage, however it may be used both in small amounts internally and is highly recommend aromatically.

27) MELISSA
Melissa officinalis
How many times have you heard a recommendation to drink lemon balm tea as an important holistic plant medicinal? Lemon balm is Melissa officinalis. From the mint family, this steam distilled herb comes from the leaves and flowers of the plant. This is a highly adulterated essential oil, generally with Lemongrass essential oil for the geranial and neral compounds. This is because it has a huge variance in properties depending on its growing environment. It is

very hard to find a farm that can produce enough high quality Melissa to maintain the supply demand.

Melissa officinalis is very similar in those important chemical properties that we find also in Lemongrass, Copaiba and Ylang Ylang. However with Melissa it is almost as if you have combined Lemongrass, Copaiba and Ylang Ylang into one powerful blend. Please make sure that this oil comes from a highly transparent supply chain if you desire true Melissa officinalis. Like Lemongrass this is an Aliphatic Aldehyde, although it holds far more Sesquiterpenes. Melissa essential oil has smaller amounts of electrophilicity than Lemongrass, yet can still be highly conductive.

Melissa supports the detoxification pathways by activating phase II enzymes, and thus protecting cells from chemical gene expression and with elimination challenges. It also offers therapeutic immune support and aids in a healthy cell cycle. Supportive of endocrine functions, nudging along the normal release of insulin from the pancreas after you have a meal. Insulin is one of the ways that our body moves blood sugar into the cells, like a key that can open up a door to store energy for later. Melissa officinalis also stimulates lipid pathways, which for my family history is very important. I can support those aches and discomforts of both emotions and body. It can be used aromatically, diluted topically, or by adding a drop into your internal routines.

In the treatment of agitation and aggression, typical Behavioral and Psychological Symptoms of Dementia (BPSDs) of Alzheimer's disease they have researched use of aromatherapy. The most used aroma-therapeutic treatments for BPSDs in dementia have been found using Melissa officinalis and Lavandula officinalis. Historical documented use of Melissa officinalis dates back to the "Materia

Medica" in approximately 50–80 BC. The Greek philosopher, Paracelsus, called Melissa "the elixir of life." The placebo-controlled clinical trial was conducted on patients affected by severe dementia in care facilities in the UK, and reported the effect of Melissa officinalis essential oil applied as massage twice a day for 4 weeks on agitation. It was measured by the Cohen-Mansfield agitation inventory. Seventy-one out of the seventy-two participants completed the trial and results demonstrated an improvement of agitation without the occurrence of significant side effects. The fact that Melissa officinalis components can cross the blood-brain-barrier most likely plays a part in this benefit. The efficacy of lemon balm hydroalcoholic extracts rather than the essential oil is also well documented.

This oil is a fun oil to use in the winter due to its higher molecular weight and its fresh lemony scent, and its support for seasonal and environmental elements. It will remain in the air for a longer time when diffused than many other uplifting essential oil aromas. You can use it to reduce those tense holiday feelings and promote emotions of relaxation and calm.

Melissa officinalis is considered to be a Middle to Top note essential oil. Melissa officinalis has been shown to offer high amounts of rosmarinic acid, which I will talk about this more, further down in the identification guide. It's important to note that ultrasound-assisted extraction is the most effective method to retain those rosmarinic acid properties in Melissa officinalis. In steam distillation, Mentha spicata (Spearmint), proved to have the highest amounts of rosmarinic acid at almost double that of Melissa officinalis. The reason this is important is because of the anti-inflammatory, antiviral and an immune modulating properties of rosmarinic acid. The cost difference and the possibilities of adulteration are far low with Spearmint than with Melissa essential oil.

In "The Blossoming Heart: Aromatherapy for Healing and Transformation", written by Robbi Zeck, ND, he talks about how Melissa "softens extreme emotions, eases resentment, gladdens the heart and engages the soul". I think that is where the benefit of Melissa officinalis lies. When working on blockages in the Sacral, Heart and Third Eye Chakras, we need to find soft, gladdening ease. When my daughter was struggling with anxiety her ND recommended lemon balm tea daily, and I thought it was interesting that the Taoists enjoyed lemon balm tea daily. Lemon balm was also cultivated by nuns and other monks in ancient record from both Norway and Central Europe. I find that this combination with as needed aromatherapy is a great source of comfort at our home.

28) MYRRH

Commiphora myrrha

One of those quoted "ancient essential oils" that is often talked about, but not often understood. Created from Myrrh Resin (the dried sap) similarly to Frankincense, true Myrrh is bitter and very high in Sesquiterpenes. Its name actually comes from the Hebrew word for bitter, "murr". It is important to know if you are getting Commiphora myrrha, or sweet Commiphora erythraea, or even Commiphora wightii which is Indian Guggul.

The Italian bitter herbal liqueur created by Bernardino Branca, *Fernet Branca*, uses Myrrh. It has been compared to a black licorice-flavored Listerine. Doesn't that sound yummy? However this was created a naturopathic medicine, and in the 19th century it was taken for a variety of reasons. Chicago craft brewery, Forbidden Roots, has creates a mimic of this liquor called Fernetic, and imperial black ale. And if you head over to Argentina you can order a Fernet con Cola, Fernet with Coca Cola. As a society we really enjoy drinking weird things, but maybe there is more to it.

The British Herbal Pharmacopoeia has recommended using Myrrh "topically for wounds and abrasions. Specifically indicated for mouth ulcers, gingivitis and pharyngitis." Several anticancer studies have been looking at the ability of Myrrh in inhibiting tumor growth. A study in 2010 concluded that Myrrh offers potent antioxidant benefits, and may protect the liver from lead poisoning. It was tested to aid in reducing bad bacteria in the mouth, and it is often used in natural mouthwashes. Traditional Chinese Medicine uses it as a drying and astringent agent, complimenting Frankincense.

It is interesting to note studies using Myrrh to see how it affects the opioid receptors in the brain. We have an opioid epidemic in this country, and a clinical study suggesting that chemicals in myrrh interact with the brain's opioid receptors to reduce pain, and we aren't doing anything about.

Commiphora myrrha will have a direct impact on every chakra except for the Heart Chakra and the Third Eye Chakra. This is Earthly oil. It is all about the emotions that ground us to this reality, and that represent our basic needs. Finances, food, self-expression, a connection to a higher power and even sexuality can all be addressed with Myrrh aroma. If you're living in a higher real of energy, and your body is falling apart, using this essential aroma may help bring your two worlds together and sync your body to your creation center.

Commiphora myrrha be used topically, aromatically, and even in a drop in a vegetable capsule when working with your practitioner.

29) MYRTLE

Myrtus communis

I love Myrtus communis for all of the balancing properties is provides. High in Monoterpenes (a-Pinene), and Oxides (1,8 Cineole), the leaves of this evergreen shrub are steam distilled. Both the Green and the Red Myrtle are called Myrtus communis, although the Green is less available than the Red is. Carrying a light aroma, it has many similar properties of Frankincense, at a fairly more affordable price point.

Myrtle is used a lot during seasonal discomforts to help return normal respiratory system functions. It also is a great anti-inflammatory for your skin blends, but the benefit in using it in your skin care is that is also can help normalize hormone imbalances. I often will recommend Myrtle communis over Salvia sclarea since Clary Sage is a uterine stimulant. However, note that Clary Sage will connect more with the underlying emotions of the Third Eye Chakra, and Myrtle with that of the Heart Chakra even though both work with these two chakra centers to promote expansive energies.

One of my favorite Jewish holidays, is Sukkot, or the Feast of Tabernacles, or simple, The Feast. It celebrates the end of the years that the Jewish people spent in the desert on their way to the Promised Land. It is means to celebrate the way in which God protected them under these difficult conditions. Part of this holiday is dwelling in a sukkah, which is a hut or a booth roofed with vegetation. In Israel the hut is often still adorned with Myrrh branches and leaves.

You may rub this oil, diluted, onto your neck to create stillness in your emotional overload of cellular confusion. You can also rub some oil on the feet at night to help relax into the sleep we need. You can add a drop into a capsule and take internally, or diffuse this oil at any time you need that body-spirit reconnect.

30) NUTMEG

Myristica fragrans

Nutmeg is the ingredient in some specialty root beers that make my daughter and I both just cringe. Just not our thing. These steam distilled seeds are mostly monoterpenes, and I have many other monoterpenes I love to select for my own aroma use. That is an important factor of selection in essential oils, which is, make sure that the oil is in sync with the clients. Today it is mostly used in those culinary products, but it has many relaxing properties just like other high Monoterpene oils. You can soothe your mind and body, and help support normal flow in the Ki of the body providing normal circulatory and digestive support.

Nutmeg essential oil contains a small amount of phenol methyl eugenol and safrole. This makes me nervous because these two have both been investigated "reasonably anticipated to be a human carcinogen." In a 2002 National Toxicology Program, ninety-eight percent of the two hundred six adults tested for methyl eugenol had detectable concentrations in their blood.

In another study when volunteers fasted overnight and then ate 12 gingersnaps that were high in methyl eugenol, it took two hours for the spiked levels to return to the fasting concentrations. We know that safrole is a known carcinogen, and so even at just an under ten percent of the composition, it makes me nervous. So although you can use

Nutmeg essential oil topically and internally, I recommend you only use this oil aromatically and in small amounts. There are many more essential oils that you can choose from to support digestion, circulatory function and chakra balance. I use the precautionary rules and always use caution in the oils that are in your cupboard.

31) ORANGE

Citrus × sinensis

Oranges, aren't they just invigorating? Of course being a citrus oil this is a cold pressed oil from the fruit peel. In an orange that is also where the greatest nutrients are. I love that my daily whole food powders include orange peel for the highly dense and vibrationally raising nutrients. Orange essential oil is high in limonene, b-myrcene and a-pinene as a high Monoterpene essential oil. During a randomized clinical trial using Orange essential oil as aromatherapy during labor, the aroma lowered their anxiety more than double that of the women in the non-aromatherapy control group. Similarly in children at the dentist office, using the Orange essential oil again as aromatherapy reduced the salivary cortisol and pulse rate due to the reduction in anxicty symptoms.

Citrus × sinensis oil creates joy. It brings up those happy moments in your life, even in children. It's very heart centric, and it opens up possibilities, energetic direction, and changes perception with just a little inhalation. It is also a really great addition when choosing an oil to add to a homemade cleaner. Who doesn't need a little pick me up when wiping down the bathroom counters? 1996 study in India, found Orange essential oil to be effective against twenty-two strains of bacteria, gram-negative and gram-positive. So maybe if you add a drop into your hand sanitizer you will find a little happier cleansing as part of your daily routine.

Oranges, aren't they just invigorating? Of course as a citrus oil this is a cold pressed oil from the fruit peel. In an orange that is also where the greatest nutrients are. I love that my daily whole food powders include orange peel for the highly dense, and vibrationally raising nutrients as there is so much more to the whole fruit than we have given it credit for.

Citrus × sinensis essential oil is high in limonene, b-Myrcene and a-Pinene as a high Monoterpene essential oil. During a randomized clinical trial using Orange essential oil as aromatic therapy during labor, women using the aromatherapy lowered their anxiety more than double that of the women in the control group. Similarly in children at the dentist office, using the Orange essential oil again as aromatherapy reduced the salivary cortisol and pulse rate due to the reduction in anxiety symptoms.

Citrus oil creates joy. It brings up those happy moments in your life, even in children. It is a very heart centric oil, that opens up possibilities, energetic direction, and changes perception with just a little inhalation.

Also this oil was studied in India in 2010 against twelve fungal strains. What they found what that it was effective against all twelve strains, completely inhibiting aflatoxin B1 which is a poisonous and cancer-causing chemical caused by mold. I started writing about aflatoxin on my blog and social media several years ago. This is an extremely potent carcinogen and major cause of mitochondria damage, thereby having the potential to negatively affect all bodily processes including skeletal muscles. Aflatoxins are found in molds that contaminate corn, rice, soybeans, and different nuts. Have you read a label lately? You'll find at least one of those in just about every packaged product in the grocery store.

Another very amazing study was in 2008 where Japanese researchers had participants walk in the forest for two to four hours. During this time they breathed in the phytochemicals that we find in both Orange essential oil and conifer oils. This activity increased their number of natural killer T-cells, and the levels of anti-cancer proteins. This was in just three days and the effects lasted for up to seven days after the trip into the forest. I have talked to you about the power of nature, and not just inhalation but getting out into it. We are born to breathe, and we are born for nature. If you can't get out into it when the weather isn't cooperating or if you don't live near a conifer forest, try aromatherapy to see how it makes you feel. When that doesn't work, you can also add a drop into a capsule to encourage metabolic function, and you can dilute for topical use, although it is phototoxic and most people do not use it in this manner.

32) OREGANO

Origanum vulgare

Do you love pizza? You may be a lover of oregano if you dream of Italian food. It is important to always keep in mind while trying to conceive that Oregano essential oil is an oil you should not use when pregnant or nursing. I always say if you are not to use something while pregnant, then don't use when trying to get pregnant as you won't know the moment of conception. This oil causes mucosal irritation. Once when my daughter was about five, she had a wart on her finger. We were using Frankincense on her every night. At this time I also was struggling with several adrenal fatigue and one a night when I could barely keep my eyes open, I grabbed the Oregano essential oil on accident. When she then started drying off from the shower, she screamed because her body started to burn. Although we don't think of essential oils and water mixing, the water can actually help the oil spread. I threw her in the cold shower while I ran to grab a jar of coconut oil to slather her with and dilute the oil down. Do not play around with this essential oil.

Origanum vulgare is steam distilled from the flowers and the buds, which may make you wonder why it's so toxic. It is important to remind yourself that just because something is natural, doesn't mean it is safe. However, Oregano does have a space in the essential oil practice, and is one of the more clinically tested oils. It has been clinically tested against antifungals because of the high Phenol properties, carvacrol and thymol which are actually Phenolic Monoterpenes. Carvacrol has been studied as effective as chlorine to wash salmonella off grape tomatoes. Wouldn't you rather buy a carvacrol washed food than chlorine washed food? This natural substance did not alter the nutritional or antioxidant value of the tomatoes, nor the look or taste.

If we look further into studies where Origanum vulgare was used against extensive antimicrobial activity, this essential oil has been used against more than food spoilage. Oregano is being used against pathogenic fungi, bacteria and yeast. Perhaps this is why we often see Oregano in oral health products, and why this Medium or Base note oil can create such a difference in these low vibrational energies that take hold in our Solar Plexus Chakra. This aroma is a foundation oil. What that means is that when you are struggling in the lower ranges of your chakra systems, which happen a lot in those high vibrational beings, you need to reconnect to the Root Chakra, Sacral Chakra and Solar Plexus Chakra systems. These three systems are where low vibrations take hold and cause some major body issues.

Consider where these chakras lie. Solar Plexus lies in the area of digestion. Everything we are being told about disease is being taken back to the gut brain today. Also dealing with those assimilation muscles responsible for the movement of digested food molecules into the cells of the body where they are used. When you balance this chakra it allows you to take back not only your personal power, but gives you the increase of nutrients for the entire body, and the hormones that work all the way up to the Third Eye Chakra. We are so interconnected, that it is important to understand it isn't all about intelligence and wisdom. Our body is deeply intuitive throughout.

As an example, your Sacral Chakra will deal with the Lumbar Plexus, which is a group of nerves that form what is called the largest nerve bundle in our plexus. A plexus is the electrical junction box in your body, and so it is wired to different parts of your body via the spinal nerves. The Sacral Plexus is connected to our feet, calves, thighs, sexual organs, buttocks and pelvis. How interesting that it lies physically lower than the Lumbar Plexus in the body, which connects to the calves, knees, thighs, groin, back and abdomen. These two areas are so interconnected they are called the Lumbosacral Plexus. This means if you impact the one, you impact the other. And as you work on your Sacral Chakra you work on your Solar Plexus. The Sacra Chakra, when balanced, will help you with elimination of emotional blocks, but also open you up to love which is opening up the Heart Chakra.

Our Root Chakra is also connected into that Lumbosacral Plexus, and yet what I found the most interesting is that it is the area most connected to our fight or flight response. If you are struggling with adrenal issues, sometimes it is better to try to work with an energetic aroma for grounding needs rather than looking at using a metabolic oil in the Throat Chakra. Oregano would be a good addition to a blend that connects to the high circadian chakras to really open up to some of those deeply rooted generational survival blockages.

33) PEPPERMINT

Mentha × piperita

The first three oils that most people use, because they are the first three oils that the top direct marketing companies share with people, are Lemon, Lavender and Peppermint essential oils. People use Mentha × piperita for so many reasons, and yet know so little about it. The two most prominent compounds in Mentha x piperita are menthol and menthone. This oil is steam distilled from the peppermint leaves, and is high in Ketones, Monoterpenols and Oxides.

Ketones, as I have spoken about before, have some dangers associated with them to those that are triggered neurotoxically. Any essential oil that is high in Ketones and Phenols can also be dangerous to our cats that metabolize essential oils in a different way than we do. Even in humans these oils are very resistant to metabolizing and can go through the body without much change in their composition.

Personally, Peppermint oil was a life saver for me when they stopped created the original Kaopectate medication in the early 90s when I was suffering with IBD. Doctors now recommend that when you have the IBD cramping or spasms to take enteric-coated capsules of peppermint oil between meals to relieve this component of inflammatory bowel disease. This was something I had to figure out for myself. However I am so glad that it exists, but it was because of that internal use that the importance of knowing about my oils and where they came from initially really started to matter for me.

Peppermint essential oil should be diluted at no more than a two percent introduction, and should not be used in bathing. The worst essential oil use I see today is in moms that are adding peppermint oil to their child's bath water when they have a fever. It will not only drop the body temperature, but drop it so fast it can create shock in the system. Peppermint is a very powerful, and what we call at my house "spicy" oil. Because of that I often recommend Spearmint as an oil option for those that want the benefits of Peppermint essential oil without some of the dangers. For those with cardiac fibrillations, you want to avoid Mentha x piperita, or if you are lacking the glucose-6-phosphate dehydrogenase (G6PD) enzyme. This mutation causes red blood cells to break down in response to certain infections, stressors or in response to certain medications, like Peppermint essential oil.

When you are using this top note energetically it will mostly be to increase your awareness within the Third Eye Chakra, and allow you to have better understanding of the knowledge you are downloading via the Third Eye. Another reason to add Peppermint oil to your blend would be in order to cool emotions with the Heart Chakra connection, and I recommend thinking about that when working with clients. You want to know what they are dealing with outside of the four walls of the session to make the most supportive aroma you can. Often you will hear the recommendation to use this oil for increasing your internal energy, and that is an option although I prefer the aroma of citrus or a woodsy aroma for that instance.

If you apply Peppermint to your hands, wash them thoroughly with a carrier oil added to break it down. Otherwise you risk what I term as "Peppermint Eye", which burns like the Dickens and requires a lot of carrier oil applied to your closed eye in hopes of removing it.

34) PATCHOULI

Pogostemon cablin

In India, over 150 tons of Pogostemon cablin is imported annually, which is fifteen times the output that the India produces. In order to increase production, the human energy-healing model was used on the plants where they found different amazing benefits at each stage of the Pogostemon cablin production. What they found was that not only were the plants healthier in appearance, but they grew taller quicker and the leaves showed a difference in features. Under the microscope it was revealed that these plants had deeper veins on the leaves with more glandular hairs on the upper side of the leaves and much larger numbers of the pores used in gaseous exchange, called stomata. The stomata are essential for the maintenance of photosynthetic activity. Now, is this something that would just work with the Patchouli plant? We don't know for sure, but I doubt it. However, I wanted to share this because it is important to understand that the care and treatment of the plants that create your oil, impacts the oil that you are using.

When researching Pogostemon cablin, they found that the twenty-six compounds in patchouli oil offered not only multi-targeted effects due to each composition, but each had strong antimicrobial effects. This oil is widely used in Traditional Chinese Medicine in dozens of formulations because of these properties for both the essential oil value and its broad range of therapeutic effects. If we look at folk medicine, Patchouli has been used to reduce fevers, chronic fatigue, restore system function, and improve the digestion. It is also often used in skin blends due to the ability to reduce minor skin irritation, and support skin restoration.

I am probably not alone in thinking that Pogostemon cablin makes me think of my hippie days. However ten gallons of Patchouli was buried with King Tut in his tomb. In the 1800s, Indian shawls and fabrics were scented with patchouli oil. Oriental fabric exporters scented their fabrics with Patchouli to repel moths, and as it happens, hippies were just attracted to the Oriental fabrics. In the late 80s, "Like A Prayer ", the album from Madonna, was packaged with patchouli oils because "she wanted to create a flavor of the '60s and the church." Interesting that it is a very powerful oil when connecting to our energetic source. This medium note oil is steam distilled from the leaves, and the older it gets, the better is smells. This oil will work from your Root Chakra to your Crown Chakra, and is Auric enhancing.

35) ROMAN CHAMOMILE

Chamaemelum nobile

While this essential oil may feel new to many of us, Chamaemelum nobile is actually an old herbal medicinal. Roman Chamomile is a very high Ester oil that is one of the oldest used herbs in the history of medicine. Chamaemelum nobile is a member of the daisy family, steam distilled from those flower petals, and it is most used to reduce anxiety and general depression.

A recent study found that chamomile flavonoids and essential oils penetrate below the skin surface into the deeper skin layers. Consider then this mediator of inflammation, Prostaglandin E(2), which is seen in diseases such as rheumatoid arthritis and osteoarthritis. Clinical studies are showing that one of Roman Chamomile anti-inflammatory activities involves the inhibition of LPS-induced prostaglandin E(2) release. Lipopolysaccharides (LPS) are an endotoxin that is present inside of a bacterial cell. When the cell disintegrates it is released. Endotoxins is thought to be the secret clue in autoimmune disorders, and so I think you will be hearing more about this in the next few years. If we look at clinical studies that target stress induced endotoxemia and low-grade inflammation, and then consider what you now know about aromatherapy, you can see the importance. Chamaemelum nobile is often used in skin formulations, due to those anti-inflammatory properties.

As an Ester, I love to consider Roman Chamomile as an alternative to Wintergreen or Birch for your topical blends for the calming and restful support to our body, and a safer oil to use with children. If you think about the use of this oil, it makes sense that this is a wonderful aroma to use for your Heart Chakra imbalances. Opening your heart can often be a simple tool to release some of the miscommunications in our cellular body.

What is even better is that this essential oil can work to align the grounding and the elevating chakras in your body. You can use this oil to increase your inner peace and intuitive nature, while being highly grounded and able to release those feelings of guilt and sorrow that often get trapped in our pancreas, Sacral Chakra. I love using this oil with energy and quantum work since emotions have such an impact on our physical body through the imbalances in our energy body field.

You can add a drop of properly tested Roman Chamomile oil into your herbal tea, use diluted topically or my favorite way is to place in your aroma diffuser or necklace. Make sure you consider this oil to expand your vision, and open yourself up to what possibilities are on your horizon waiting for acknowledgement.

36) ROSEMARY

Rosmarinus officinalis

Rosemary essential oil is an aroma that although used a lot in complementary therapies, can increase the risk of seizures in those sensitive to its neurotoxic properties. With this knowledge you can sense that it is very stimulating and high in Monoterpene properties, but it is the Ketones that are the trigger. Do not use this oil when trying to conceive, pregnant or nursing.

This steam distilled herb works a lot in the Throat and Heart Chakra. If we consider discussing the Plexuses, the Cervical Plexus and Brachial Plexus connect the Throat and Heart Chakras, as well as have a deep connection into the Cardiac Plexus. The Cardiac Plexus is deeply connected in front of the trachea. Your Brachial Plexus begins at the back of the neck, then, and extends into our armpit. The Cervical Plexus is more of a supportive plexus that runs through the muscles, blood vessels and sensory branches of the neck, throat, scalp and occipital regions. And of course the vagus nerve starts in the brainstem, and is connected to all of the plexus bundles in our bodies, and I have only touched on a few.

So when you select an oil to raise your mental activity, maybe you can consider a different Base note, like Copaiba essential oil, and blend it with a Top or Middle note that works with what you are going for, like citrus oil. It offers some of the similar support to memory as Rosemary essential oil, and yet does not contain the side effects that you may find with it.

There is a lot of antibacterial research on Rosmarinus officinalis, which is why we see it used in foods, medicine and cosmetics as a preservative. It is high in rosmarinic acid and carnosic acid which is the components that can prevent oils and fats from becoming rancid. We talked about the anti-inflammatory, antiviral and immune modulating properties of rosmarinic acid before. There are other high rosmarinic acid oils that I prefer over Rosemary. However, when you are working with a topical formulation using high omega-6 fatty acids, you may want to use Rosemary in it for the preservation properties. However label your product accordingly because so many people do not know the dangers that lurk in this oil.

This oil is often used topically when well diluted, or to purify the air aromatically. As well it is added to dishes after cooking for flavor.

38) SCOTCH PINE

Pinus sylvestris

Perhaps the aroma is the reason I felt so at home the moment I drove under the bridge and into the Seattle area. I adore pine trees, and the aroma after a rain storm in the Pacific Northwest is like you are standing alone in the middle of the forest. If you remember that the Japanese found that just walking in the forest can boost our natural killer t-cell activity. Hippocrates first used pine tree oils for respiratory support, and the Romans use it in ritual and religious ceremonies. Native Americans used the pine needles as a pest repellent, and made the needles into tea to relieve the body in a similar way to Hippocrates methods.

Scotch Pine essential oil is mostly composed of a-Pinene. In 2015 Pinus sylvestris needle extract and essential oil was found to suppress the viability of several human cancer cell lines showing some selectivity to estrogen receptor negative breast cancer cells. In fact in another study mice kept in a fragrant environment enriched with a-Pinene show reduced melanoma growth. A-Pinene is found in many essential oils, not just Pinus sylvestris. It can be found in Juniperus communis and Eucalyptus globulus. So again, you can choose an oil with similar properties and create a blend that offers what you desire. I love to include a-Pinene for short-term memory support, to support our normal inflammatory response and open the airways so you have improved airflow to breathe.

Scotch Pine is also high in terpinolene, which offers some unique wellness benefits. This offers the sedative properties of pine, and has a depressant action on our central nervous system. This offers a wonderful aroma for those that have high functioning brains that do not want to turn off, and the anxious feelings often associated with it. This is an abundant Terpene in cannabis.

This oil can oxidize quicker than others, and should be sure to store in a cool, dark space. If you are grounded, and open and still feeling out of balance, Scotch Pine can balance the Sacral, Solar Plexus, Heart and Throat Chakras to allow the energy to flow in a more expansive manner. It will declutter your chakra fields, and can be used for many reasons associated with each of these chakra zones. Do not use this essential oil internally, even though you may have made pine tea before. If can irritate mucosa, cause nausea, vomiting, diarrhea, trigger migraines and create dizziness. I do not use this oil with women that are trying to conceive, are pregnant or nursing.

39) SPEARMINT

Mentha spicata

Remember when we talked about the anti-inflammatory, antiviral and immune modulating properties of rosmarinic acid? My favorite clinical study of rosmarinic acid has been in its use to protect against seasonal and environmental elements. In a landmark original research article, extracts containing rosmarinic acid were shown to be an effective treatment for humans suffering from seasonal allergic rhinoconjunctivitis.

In this 21-day, double-blind, placebo-controlled, randomized, age-matched parallel group study, patients with seasonal allergic rhinoconjunctivitis were given a total daily dose of either 50 mg or 200 mg of rosmarinic acid and kept a daily diary of their symptoms. I like to use Spearmint over Rosemary every day of the week.

Weight can vary with essential oils but the average essential oil is 20 drops per gram. Mentha spicata was tested to have almost 60 mg of rosmarinic acid per gram in a comparative study of rosmarinic acid content in some plants of Labiatae family. Twenty drops would be far too much of any essential oil for someone to use, and you have to remember that is a comparison of a supplemental dose and an essential oil component. You should never look at a clinical study and try to recreate the dosage on your own, and instead work with your doctor, pharmacist and Aromatherapist to determine the best use of any essential oil.

With Mentha spicata, I would recommend as an alternative to try diffusing some Spearmint essential oil as it is mild enough to be used around children for that seasonal and environmental protection. In the clinical study, two groups of students were tested against this aromatherapy support. Group One nebulized a mix of saline and Citrus sinensis oil, while the other group nebulized a mix of saline and Mentha spicata. After the lung tests were performed they found that both groups of students showed an improvement in their breathing after using the oils. Use of the oils also significantly reduced how long it took the students to run the same distance, even without using the oils. Don't overlook the benefits of Spearmint.

I will occasionally use a drop of Spearmint internally to support my digestive system in a similar way to Peppermint as it promotes digestive function. But I prefer to use Spearmint aromatically, and will never use topically without high dilution rates.

40) SPRUCE

Picea mariana

This is considered the Black Spruce, and it works just like it sounds. Steam distilled from the needles it is a grounded essential oil. A very gorgeous essential oil to use in your aroma routine around the holidays, this oil has come to be one of my favorite oils to add to my aromatherapy necklace year round. While it is similar in aroma to other pines or fir tree oils, it is one of the most versatile oils in this area. High in Esters and Monoterpenes, for someone that doesn't love citrus or floral aromas; you can instead use the Picea mariana aroma in a blend for the restorative and stabilizing effects. I find that this oil has the most in common with Cedarwood essential oil in its healing properties.

Decades ago this resin was used as like our chewing gum is today, and for respiratory support as mostly a spruce needle tea. It provides your simple immune support, and I love to use it when the body is creating too much. When you think of too much, have too much mucus, too much cortisol, and too much energy, this is when your body is calling for the support of Picea mariana.

Diluted, this is a great oil to rub on the back just above the kidneys to help support some of that tension and anxious feelings. You can use it to help slip into bedtime relaxation, and yet when used during the day it will increase your alertness. The bark of the Spruce is rich in bioactive polyphenols, although I have seen very little bark essential oil and instead think we will see this increasing as a powdered supplement. Santalum austrocaledonicum is another favorite bark essential oil, and an alternative you can consider if you do not have Spruce in your cupboard.

When you are working with any client that has a struggle with grounding, and remaining connected to the Earth, I would recommend you add Picea mariana to your sessions. This oil will not only pull their connection back into the Earth realm, but it will open up the Heart chakra to increase the release of energy blocks in the fourth chakra. So often, those of us that choose to live in the higher realms do so because of emotional pain that we have had in our life. This makes us very tuned in to be able to help others, but leaves us with broken bodies unable to ground and connect to what the Earth provides.

Several clinical studies have looking into the impact of grounding on those that suffer with autoimmune disorders, and other diseases, especially in what we call Earthing. Grounding improves your sleep, normalizes our cortisol patterns to establish the optimal circadian rhythm. As this improves, there are a number of others benefits that can be seen. Research showed an improvement in muscle recovery, and delayed soreness. What they believe is happening is that the Earth sends mobile electrons into the body which act as natural antioxidants. This energy is semi-conducted through the connective tissue matrix, including through the inflammatory barricade if one is present, which can neutralize reactive oxygen species and other oxidants in the repair field. ROS is reactive molecules containing oxygen in the body which in theory can damage lipid, DNA, RNA, and proteins, contributing to the physiology of aging. As such, grounding can protect healthy tissue from damage.

Spruce is high in camphene. This property offers a soothing effect on our nerves to help support our body's natural inflammatory response to stress. A lesser known terpenoid, it has powerful benefits that we are just beginning to understand. It stands out as a powerful oil to use in skin blends and could offer a combined mind and body support system when used in this way.

I have not used Spruce internally other than as I would Tea Tree for a mouthwash ingredient. I find that it works best when it is used aromatically or topically for relief of a sour body and mind.

41) SWEET BASIL

Ocimum basilicum

Sweet Basil, steam distilled from the leaves and flowering tops of one of my favorite plants. It is no wonder as it is high in Monoterpenols. This top note is a nice addition to a focusing blend, although it can take over the blend if you tip your hand too heavily. If you are looking for safer stimulating oils, this may be the oil you desire.

Ocimum basilicum is often compared to Ocimum sanctum, also known as Holy Basil. However Holy Basil grows larger than Sweet Basil, and can tolerate a narrower soil ph. than Sweet Basil. Sweet Basil essential oil was tested alongside Holy Basil essential oil, and what they found was that Ocimum basilicum showed a greater effect in the disruption of biofilm. In most of their activity the results were similar. However with both of these there is a concern to make sure that there is a concentration limit for alkenylbenzenes. The toxicity of alkenylbenzenes has been found to be relatively low, especially when you are eating sweet basil. However it is still considered to have tumorigenic, capable of forming tumors, potential. So you should consider this when using an essential oil such as Sweet Basil, and do not overdo it.

Sweet Basil can be supportive of opening up the Heart Chakra, and expanding your Crown Chakra energy waves to clarify your thoughts and calm when we are feeling energetically awake. This oil can also be very supportive in the astral plane, and will protect against negative energies. This oil has been used internally, aromatically and with dilution topically. Find the way that it works best for you.

42) SWEET FENNEL

Foeniculum vulgare

If you ask anyone there is a high use of Sweet Fennel for digestive support, to relieve flatulence, or to help patients with chronic constipation in the essential oil and supplemental industry. We often see fennel added to digestive blends, used for its balancing hormonal properties, or in a topically cream to help reduce sore muscles. Oral essential fennel oil in capsules and fennel extract in vaginal cream have long both been used to improve symptoms in postmenopausal women with daily use. It is also often used for hormonal support to promote lactation, and promote menstruation. It has even been used for increasing the male libido. Such a simple essential oil, and yet so little about these full properties is known or talked about in the aroma community.

On the one hand there are some studies that showcase that Foeniculum vulgare can go to work against H. pylori, where many drugs fail. But when we consider that Foeniculum vulgare contains mostly anethole, it starts to become concerning. One problem is in the anethole is very skin sensitive and having estrogen-like effects. A study using rats with anethole revealed some non-neoplastic and neoplastic lesions in the older rats, although mostly reduced weight gain with the highest dosage. Anethole is a reproductive hormone modulator, and several hours after taking it internally in these mice it was still found in the stomach. The same properties, though, have made it studied for its anti-inflammatory abilities working on the same pathways at Celebrex.

The other problem is the small amounts of estragole, recently show to have carcinogenicity, now requires that fennel has been charged to be dangerous for humans especially if used as a seed decoction for babies. In just two weeks breastfed newborns appear to have toxicity from drinking fennel tea, which has far small amounts of these properties than the essential oil does. It has been categorized by the State of California as a carcinogen for almost two decades. It has been found to cause transgene mutations in animals, and what I found while doing my aroma studies is that avocado is even more toxic having far higher levels of estragole than fennel seeds do. Another high estragole herb is tarragon.

Sweet Fennel oil is very often an adulterated essential oil, which can create an even more toxic oil. Use of this oil should be cautioned in those on diabetic medication or anticoagulants. It should be avoided if you have endometriosis and estrogen-dependent cancers. Also if you have peptic ulcers, hemophilia or other bleeding disorders, or are preparing to undergo surgery as it inhibits platelet aggregation.

The possibility that Foeniculum vulgare is potentially carcinogenic, and yet still being used by breastfeeding moms leaves me with a lot of concerns. It is a lipophilic essential oil, which can easily cross cell membranes by free diffusion. Foeniculum vulgare is also considered genotoxic, and is an oil that can trigger seizures. Well most oil companies offer this oil to be used internally, aromatically and topically, I am not one to recommend it until there have been further studies about the way this oil functions with the human body, and due to the high level of synthetic adulterations. There are so many other oils that will work for the Sacral and Solar Plexus Chakras, including Ginger, which has so many better possible uses than Fennel for digestive support.

43) TANGERINE

Citrus reticulata

Who doesn't love the smell of a freshly peeled tangerine? Like all citrus essential oils this oil is both uplifting, and phototoxic. However, when dealing with children or those holding onto childhood trauma, Citrus reticulata can offer aromatic happiness. If one citrus fruit was put in the dictionary to showcase happiness, it would be the tangerine. Tangerine essential oil works so well as an inhaled aroma that is often used in cleaners. I love to use it to cleanse a space before doing energy work, not just for the purification but because it opens us up to feelings. Intuitive work is often an energetic relationship that is part empathic. When you get a massage from a therapist that just knows where you need the manipulative release, and you don't have to say a word, that is the empathic knowing.

It may be surprising that tangerine trees are native to China, as many of us may consider the essence of a tangerine to come from some tropical paradise. When working with children, I move away from Tangerine because even with dilution it can cause an irritation if you desire to use it topically. Being a far more skin sensitive essential oil, I often will grab instead for a Green Mandarin, which is an essential oil cold pressed from the unripe mandarin peel. Oils within the same note class, and even being similar in coming from fruit peels, can have so many differing properties to choose from.

Consider that the skin of the tangerine is a much darker, almost reddish orange color as compared to the ripe mandarin. That skin color is a natural sign of the essential oil properties. The richer color offers more grounding and sensual properties than the mandarin does. As well, the tangerine skin has a bumpy, defined texture, whereas the mandarin is smooth. I look at this as the goosebumps of the energetic Citrus reticulata oil. Goosebumps used to be connected to more of a physiologic aspect of the human body. Goosebumps make our energetic and physical being appear larger. Of course this is far more apparent on a male or me after a long winter without shaving my legs. However for most energy workers sense that feeling of goosebumps in connection to Spirit.

"Gheranda Samhita", which is a Hatha Yoga textbook, defines goosebumps as bhakti. This refers to love and devotion, attachment and faith. When we feel this physical or emotional feeling, it is a sign we are on a spiritual path. As such, I find that Tangerine is an aroma that moves us along that path, while keeping us in our truth. Zen Master Thich Nhat Hanh even has a tangerine meditation, and he says, "Each time you look at a tangerine, you can see deeply into it. You can see everything in the universe in one tangerine. When you peel it and smell it, it's wonderful. You can take your time eating a tangerine and be very happy."

Tangerine is often used in massage blends because of the sedative properties as well as the lymphatic detoxifying abilities due to its support of our normal circulatory function. So you can dilute and use topically, take in a small amount internally, or use this aromatically to create your own clear energy path.

44) TEA TREE
Melaleuca alternifolia

This is another oil that you either love, or you don't. Although it is often compared to Melaleuca quinquenervia viridiflora, they are very different. I personally am not a fan of the aroma of MQV essential oil, and prefer Melaleuca alternifolia or even Leptospermum scoparium if I can find a good source. This steam distilled oil comes from mostly wild harvested leaves, from Australia. It is a relatively high costing aroma, and as such as much a three quarters of all Tea Tree oils on the market are thought to be adulterated. Just this fall new laboratory guidance was released to help distributors to assess the authenticity of their Tea Tree oil.

Melaleuca alternifolia is widely sought after due to its antimicrobial properties. It is used in traditional Ayurveda for healing the skin of seborrheic dermatitis, infections and burns. It has also been tested for use of human parasitic infection of the gastrointestinal tract caused by the consumption of raw or undercooked seafood containing larvae. Anisakis simplex has been implicated in gastric, intestinal, and allergic clinical disorders, and as with many other infections there is a demand for natural products due to the development of resistance to our pharmaceuticals.

My first experience with Tea Tree oil was in a skincare product for creating smaller pores and reducing acne. This is a wonderful oil to use with a carrier when you are dealing with a histamine based skin reaction, like with the keto rash. However my two favorite uses of Melaleuca alternifolia are to use on my gums after brushing, and to apply at the base of my nasal pathway to promote normal respiratory function. I have only once taken Tea Tree internally to promote a return to a normal immune function when I was struggling during the winter season. You can also just add a drop to a cotton ball and place the cotton ball at the entry to your inner ear.

This oil is about half Monoterpenes and half Monoterphenols. Remember that the Monoterphenols are very skin friendly essential oils, where Monoterpenes are the more fragrant anti-inflammatory constituents. As either a Top or Middle Note oil, this oil is very good at connecting and balancing those lower chakra meridians. Your Root Chakra is always active with regards to your meridians. If we think about the Nadis, the channels through which, in traditional Indian medicine and spiritual science, the energies of the physical body, the subtle body and the causal body are said to flow, this is an exceptional oil to use for this work. If you remember there are 72,000 of these channels in practice in our body, although there are claims and the possibility for millions. Using this oil with your yoga practice and Kundalini breathing, it is creating a clear energy flow from below to above to keep the Ki flowing through the channels as it should. This is an especially important aroma to have at your disposal when you have stuck energy in your microcosmic orbit circulation. Let this be an oil to keep the spark of creation moving in your being.

It is important to note that contact dermatitis is more frequently reported with Tea Tree essential oil than many others. Do not forget to patch test with your essential oils before use. Remember when people claim toxicity, it is important to know the claims. Several oral toxicity reports have come through in recent years. One was a sixty year old man who ingested a half teaspoon of oil, followed by a dramatic rash. The other report was of a patient that drank a half of a tea cup of tea tree oil and was comatose for twelve hours and semi-conscious for another thirty-six hours. One drop is all you generally need, when a doctor, pharmacist or Aromatherapist is working with you.

45) THYME

Thymus vulgaris

There are so many ways that Thymus vulgaris has been clinically studied, which is great for having proof of the benefits available in using this oil. It has been used for centuries with both the Ancient Greek and Ancient Egyptians. This oil has high Monoterpene and lessor Phenol components, and is a steam distilled flowering herb. Its name comes from the Greek word meaning "to fumigate" which is quite fitting for its natural abilities.

Thymus vulgaris is a natural antibacterial and was even used as a possible alternative to traditional antibiotics in skin infections with rescued dogs as a topical treatment. When clinically working with Thymus vulgaris against thirty clinical isolates of oral pathogens, the agar disk diffusion showed inhibition zones around the various concentrations, and revealed a strong inhibitory activity on oral pathogens. Other studies have shown that a topical gel formulation containing essential oil of Thymus vulgaris is a promising alternative for cosmetic and phyto-therapeutic use against topical infections. Unlike Tea Tree we do not have enough long term data to showcase that the likelihood of developing strains resistant to these therapeutic agents is minimal. However it is a step in the right direction.

Another great Middle Note essential oil, that seems to work in those middle chakra realms, you can use this aromatically just as you would topically to encourage a purification of the energy body, and an energizing shot to your relationships, creativity, emotional and personal powerhouses. I admit that I don't use Thyme oil a lot in my personal practice, although it supports cellular integrity, and can be protective against oxidative stress. I will use it on occasion, mostly for those reasons both topically and internally. It is not my favorite smell, so I rarely use this oil aromatically.

It is at a high risk for creating mucosa irritation, and skin sensitization. It should not be used when bathing. This oil may inhibit blood clotting and can interact with some medications. Be sure to talk to your pharmacist before adding Thyme into your oil rotation.

46) TRUE LAVENDER
Lavandula angustifolia
Lavandula angustifolia is also called, Common Lavender. This lavender is the English lavender rather than the French lavender. English lavender is heartier, and as such I feel like it's a better fit for some people. Used mostly for calming and relaxation, it is a very soothing aroma. When you are looking to balance any overall instability, this is the better choice in my opinion. It is like the difference between the wild blueberry and the commercially grown blueberry. Both have some similarities, but you gain so much more from what the wild blueberry has been through.

Unlike the less-commonly grown French Lavendula dentata,
Lavandula angustifolia essential oil which is steam distilled from the flowers has been sold in the United States as an over-the-counter oral capsule. This is generally used for stress relief, relaxation, and support for healthy sleeping patterns. Sold generally in 60mg to 80mg, which is in line with clinical studies. This is equivalent to just one drop of True Lavender oil.

True Lavender essential oil is a very special oil for creating a different perspective on everything from relationships or emotions. It will balance those hyper energy fluctuations, even though it is stimulating oil. It can be diluted and used topically with children, although it is generally used aromatically for calming properties. Topically it can be used to moisten skin, or improve skin conditions due to bug bites, cuts and bruises. As well as it calms the mind, so it calms the spirit and the body's tension. An often forgotten oil to use when you feel like you exercise got the best of you.

47) VETIVER

Vetiveria zizanioides

This tiny little bottle of goodness sits on the ledge of my granite surround in my bathroom. Not only is it a healing oil, but it is very grounding, which I often need before heading into the traffic to take my daughter out to classes. However should we use this oil in the morning or before bed? A good portion of our nightly sleep is meant to be slow-wave sleep. So many people have these very dysfunctional sleep patterns. Most of our deep sleep is what we consider slow-wave sleep. What we need at night is rejuvenation, and what studies have found is that Vetiver inhalation significantly increases total waking time, and reduced slow-wave sleep time which means it is definitely a before mid-afternoon essential aroma. Instead this oil is the safer Rosemary, supporting our learning and memory processes. Vetiveria zizanioides, although stimulating can also be balancing for those with rapid brain patterns for reasons we will get into in a minute. This is a safe essential oil for use around children, and yes it does contain a small amount of neurotoxic Ketones. But it is mostly Sesquiterpenols and Sesquiterpenes and is not currently on my unsafe to use for those sensitive to neurotoxins list.

Additional clinical research has looked at the biological activity in the human skin cell. Vetiver was found to not only regulate gene expression, but it impacted the genes that are related to tissue remodeling and metabolism. This oil was found to have strong antiproliferative activity in these pre-inflamed human dermal fibroblast cells. Our dermal fibroblasts cells are responsible for generating connective tissue and allowing our skin to recover from injury. Though this was suspected as Vetiver is a very calming essential oil, the big surprise was the way it impacted cholesterol metabolism which means it may be a good therapeutic candidate for not just skincare, but also for obesity.

Steam distilled from the Vetiveria zizanioides root, this is your survival chakra oil. It will ground you, and support your as you are building yourself up. It promotes creation, and opens your being to a calmer meditation which can create some pretty complex changes in the physical and energetic body. ADHD is one of the most diagnosed disorders in our young children today. In fact my daughter was diagnosed with anxiety that was directly related to her ADHD. In any given classroom, up to thirty percent of the students are diagnosed with ADHD.

With ADHD there is a dominant pattern of Theta brain waves. These are the brainwaves that we see most often in our sleep, and when we meditate. Dr. Terry S. Friedmann ran a brain wave test using the aromas of Cedarwood, Lavender and Vetiver essential oils. The goal was to increase the Beta waves that show we are engaged in mental activities. Of course Lavender did nothing, which is why you use it to fall deep asleep quickly. Both Vetiver and Cedarwood increased the Beta waves by thirty-two percent and improved the brain activity, which reduced the symptoms of ADHD. Surprisingly the oil that alleviated some of the emotional symptoms in further testing was Coriander. I wish they would have tested a combination of citrus oils, Coriander, Cedarwood and Vetiver, however I recommend you try that and see how you feel. Especially knowing how Coriander can support our brain in these high EMF zones, it is worth a trial run. Just remember to go very low Coriander in your blend, with a more balanced Cedarwood, Vetiver and a citrus choice like Mandarin.

Knowing what I have learned about Vetiver, I can see why it is more balancing in the lower chakras, rather than the higher chakras. Since Theta brain waves are associated with our memories, beliefs, and restorative subconscious energies, adding in Vetiver would be like a shock to a peaceful, meditative session. This oil isn't one I would select when working with a client in an energy healing, relaxing session.

My favorite Haitian Vetiver is grown using sustainable farming and harvesting techniques. It is very difficult to harvest, as first Vetiver is grown there on hillsides. This keeps the roots from rotting as can happen in paddocks. Vetiver is very cleansing both energetically and for the area it is grown in. So it can be grown in paddocks to clean the water to support a herd of animals for a rancher. However it is not the best way to grow Vetiver for use as an essential oil.

With so many ways to use Vetiveria zizanioides, how will you choose? You can use it topically in a lotion or a homemade facial wash. You can use it aromatically to promote both a feeling of relaxation and to wake up the Theta brain. This oil has been used internally in a clinical setting and so should not be used in this manner without working with a medical provider.

48) WINTERGREEN

Gaultheria procumbens

This warming oil has a lot of misunderstandings due to the high amount of synthetics available for a variety of reasons. This oil is almost completely made up of Esters, and should not be used internally due to the potential for toxicity. This is an oil you do not want to have in reach of your children as less than 1 tsp has been implicated in the deaths of several children. This was due to high amounts of methyl salicylate, which is similar to aspirin and quickly absorbed in our gastrointestinal tract. One drop of Wintergreen is 60mg, and aspirin toxicity in an adult weighing 150 pounds has been documented at just 1.5 tsp of Wintergreen.

Where Wintergreen gets its popularity is that same methyl salicylate offers an ability to reduce sore muscles and promote fitness recovery. This oil, even for topical diluted use should not be overused. Wintergreen can inhibit blood clotting, nor used while taking anticoagulant medication. This oil should not be used when trying to conceive, pregnant or breastfeeding as it can be harmful to the embryos and the fetus. Do not use with children.

Wintergreen can be used aromatically when the Throat chakra is blocked due to energetic pain, as it will expand and uplift your truth. Do not diffuse around small children or cats as they cannot metabolize this oil in the same manner that an adult can.

50) YLANG YLANG

Cananga odorata

I have never liked the aroma of Ylang Ylang, and yet is such a valuable essential oi. Investigations done on this oil found that using this oil for aromatherapy offers relief to those suffering from depression and stress due to its calming abilities. A very balanced oil because it has a little of everything. The highest amounts of Sesquiterpenes, it also offers Esters, Monoterpenols, Phenols, Sesquiterpenols, Monoterpenes and Oxides. This is truly your full Middle Note oil, although in the right blend you can use it for your base

Ylang ylang is one of those oils that can be varied and different based on whether is a complete distillation or not. It can be used in hair formulations to help promote a thicker head of hair, and as a licensed Cosmetologist, many clients love having Ylang Ylang treatments.

An aromatic choice for an essential oil, Cananga odorata helps release tense feelings, and can be very supportive for a stressed out parent. This is because of the properties it offers for the Heart Chakra, and the Sacral Chakra which are very important for relationships, and in opening up to unconditional love. It isn't that we don't love our children unconditionally; it is just that they are children. A little Ylang Ylang in an aroma necklace or bracelet may become the secret stash in your parenting tool bag. Open up your heart, release anger, create an awareness of the gratitude you have for everything in your life. Add this to your sessions, however use caution in topical application due to skin sensitization. Do not use on children.

This is the end of the in-depth Individual Oil Identification.

12

ENTREAROMATHERAPY

Imagine two stores sitting side-by-side in a popular shopping mall. One is your go-to shop for just about everything. They sell garden tools, candy bars, T-shirts, car parts and baby bottles.

The other store is more exclusive, and the smells are amazing. In fact, the only thing they sell is chocolate. Belgian chocolate, Swiss chocolate, dark and milk chocolate, chocolate covered peanuts and chocolate flavored gummy bears. If it's chocolate, they stock it. And if it's not chocolate, you won't find It on their shelves. Just walking past the store your mouth starts to water as you inhale the aroma of the most amazing smells of joy, love, and the holidays. Now you may say, I don't want to sell chocolate, and just focusing in on one thing is limiting. Perhaps it is, but what aroma offers is something that clarifying and limbic connection that store one misses. Despite how many twenty percent off coupons they send me, I rarely buy from the popular mall store. What about you?

When you clarify and define your business offerings when thinking about essential oils, you want to make sure that what you create closely matches your business awareness and vibe. High end hotels are creating signature, mind lifting scents to keep you coming back again and again.

Langham Hotels uses a blend of green grass, rose, lily of the valley, and jasmine essential oils in their Ginger Flower room scent, and I can imagine that when you walk in you just feel the calm emotions pour out of your body. Being aware of what your niche is creates how you bring essential oils and aromatherapy into your business. You will be in a far better position to attract your ideal client when you gain a sense of clarity, and look at what aromatherapy can offer your clients. Not only that, but you'll have customers lining up to pay a premium for your services.

So now you know why the Langham Hotel is a successful elite hotel, and why customers have such an emotional connection almost as soon as they walk into their hotel and inhale the smells. Your anxiety drops and your pocketbook opens. Many hotels now offer items you can take home with you for a price, like a comfy white robe or a bottle of Ginger Flower Room Spray. As a hotel, they wouldn't have a need for a partnership with an aromatherapy company, instead working with an Aromatherapist to create a signature blend that they can manufacture, or order.

There is a spa in the Pacific Northwest that had a custom "forest scent" created to use in their spa to help the clients feel like they were out in nature as they entered. A spa may have a greater ability to offer more essential oils for their clients, but remember 'the everything' store? Share what matters, rather than sharing everything.

I say this because at first glance most people think that 'the everything' store has more traffic. The truth is that they may. This is okay because they probably have to sell a lot in order to hit profitability. Your niche business is different. You will generally have fewer customers, but the average client is far more loyal, spends more money per visit, and raves to her friends about exactly what you offer. The average client at 'the everything' store? A single rumor of a lower price at a new store across town, and he or she is gone without a backward glance.

What does this have to do with your business and aroma services or product offerings? Just everything.

If you picked up this book you are connected to a natural niche market regardless of if this is your service or product offering. So, it's critical for you to know exactly what you want to provide, and to whom. As an Aromatherapist your offering should and would be essential oils, and you would work with your clients on a more individual basis to make sure that they are getting the right oils for themselves, and their family. Your essential oil client probably does not want a hodgepodge of fitness products with no clear direction and without a cohesive brand, you may make a few sales (especially if you work cheap) but you won't gain a loyal following. You'll be like that first store, always chasing after new customers, because the old ones keep wandering away in search of a better price. While most direct sales companies offer 'the everything' store of products, the products your client is looking for is first essential oils in an easy to use manner.

If this is your business marketing plan you have a virtual storefront that doesn't educate your clients, that is what your brand becomes. You are not just working with one client at a time; you are working to educate many clients, and a team of clients and prospective team members. That means also that you have to keep in line with their brand, their regulations, or focus in on the brand of you. Aroma instantly tells a story, so does your story tell your new store or online platform visitor exactly what you do? Are your offerings priced in line with your market?

Don't be afraid to take a hard look at your current offerings and get rid of those low-priced, fringe products that are diluting your brand. Focus on the core products and services, and work to make them better and more valuable, and before you know it, your brand will have a loyal following, too.

When I Googled Instagram #essentialoils there was 5.8 million posts using that hashtag. This is a billion dollar industry, and every day a new brand is coming into play, which is why sustainability, transparent testing and knowledge of essential oils really make a difference. Manhattan moms are creating CBD infused essential oils products for women, and making a killing selling $90 kits to hundreds of moms that like many are looking for some Zen, or to curb cravings and reduce the bloat. So there are new avenues being created in the essential oil industry.

Creating your own oil brand means researching small batch wholesalers, bottling in your bathtub from giant oil containers, labeling, etc. While the payoff for creating a niche brand can be huge, the truth is that all businesses are on a cycle of start to finish. With the fast marketing of social media, your business idea today could be here today and gone tomorrow. That is why it's important to decide what the brand of you is, and then how to use aromatherapy as a funnel from some side hustle or as a part of something bigger.

Mindfulness is the future of business, and is no longer just about yoga and meditation. Mindfulness had infiltrated Fortune 500 companies and is growing like wildflowers in the biohacking communities. Self-development is out, and mindfulness is in. Mindfulness and aromatherapy go hand in hand as you have learned. You may create scents for business meetings, employee retreats, yoga studios, spas, puppy training classes and more. The ideas are endless in the congruence of aroma and mindful living. I believe that just as we are seeing meditation move into the technology sector, so will aromatherapy more and more. Plant based, nature based, technology based, minimalistic living is what is coming to your business in the future. So how will you get on board?

My personal business started as life and business coaching, but through the years it has developed through an awareness of what my soul purpose really is. I now say that my business is in the subtle body energy creation. Although through the years I have been educated in many areas and am a Certified Aromatherapist, Fitness Instructor, Personal Trainer, Life Coach and Energy Practitioner; the truth for me was that everything actually starts with the subtle body energy field. One way that I have created my niche market is in working with technology that reads the electrical signals in the body, as well as the electrical signals in the essentials to determine what body craves energetically in mind, body and soul. Using this can help me select the right essential oils or nutrients that can help a client's energy balance. My business of bringing the ideas of Traditional Chinese Medicine into practice with the biohacking technology of electromagnetic frequencies and a little intuition and knowledge to guide my clients to the right essential oils for their life targets.

Another way is by building a tribe of similarly minded friends that work with me to spread the benefits of working with essential oils, but all in their own way. When I work with other energy workers, they are often drawn to what I am doing, but not always in the same manner that I work, which is great because it creates an additional funnel of income and a space for me to be more aware of what else is possible in this vast universe. Ask you shall receive, but you have to be open to that energy. Marketing a business opportunity isn't for everyone, and you have to have the spark for that growth mindset.

If you are a fitness trainer maybe you are creating oils that help support the muscles of your clients, or as a baker maybe you want to add essential oils into your signature cupcakes. The secret to aromatherapy is that in order to keep growing a business infused with aroma; you have to make sure that is sparks something inside of your being. Boredom is one of the biggest contributors to the feeling of being stuck in a rut in our business life. Being bored is a symptom of a mind that is not fully engaged, and it can lead to complacency. Complacency blocks the congruency of energetic movement. The longer you remain unexcited about the business you're creating, the harder it can become to motivate yourself to look for ways to change. This is something that invites Shining Sparkling Syndrome where you just keep grabbing for something to stick in your business, which rarely does.

As you explore the expansion of using essential oils in your entrepreneur life, look for ways to stretch your comfort zone. Make a list of what aromatherapy can offer to your business. It can include new topics or skills you'd like to learn, types of people you'd be interested to meet, experiences that would delight you or something as simple as a different kind of food you want to try. Your list should include baby steps and large leaps. Start with the small stuff and work your way to bigger things or mix it up as the mood strikes. Select a few oils that offer a possibility for your business, and then see how they feel. Through your exposure to alternative ideas and information, you are bound to come across experiences, people and, hopefully, passions that may shift your worldview. You may begin to appreciate the simple things more and begin to focus on the joy that comes from such riches. These are the things happiness is made of, and what really creates a successful business.

Continuous learning and growing, and asking what else you can achieve and provide will offer your business a multitude of benefits. These are just a handful. Hopefully, you now have the awareness to commit yourself to your own journey of aromatherapy self-discovery.

13

CASE STUDIES

When you are working with an aromatherapy course, and not just a book, you would have case studies that you would need to create in order to pass your course. Aromatherapy is what we like to call supportive care as essential oils are not meant to be used as an Aromatherapist in diagnosis, prevention, treatment or to cure any disease and/or illness. Supportive care is using tools that help your body and soul cope with whatever is going on to help create the best quality of life. As we have discussed this often takes place due to the overwhelming ability of essential oils to target our emotional memories.

When creating your case study you will want to use an intake form to get vital information about what your client is dealing with, what supplementation and medications they are using, any illnesses they have, is the client pregnant or trying to conceive or do they suffer with epilepsy or other issues that trigger seizures, and what is your client looking for in terms of use of essential oils. Working with a client that is looking to create a facial serum is very different than working with a client that has chronic aches and pain. The one item that is the same with all of us, though, would be that we all have a current emotional state. I always consider emotions into the blending because of the relationship between mind and body.

This information can give you the basic information to start choosing oils that you think would work for your client. Let your client know that aromatherapy is a complementary therapy, and if possible let your client smell the oils you have selected to see how they respond. We all have different versions of emotional memories, but they are all tied to aroma. What makes you smile could make your client make that yucky face.

Once you are prepared to proceed, make sure you dilute the oils properly or give your client the instructions on how to dilute the essential oil or essential oil blend. When working with clients topically, make sure they understand to let you know if they have any rashes or feelings of discomfort when you apply the topical oil solution. Any oil taken internally should be offered by only a physician or Certified Aromatherapist with the proper instructions and all alternative practices should be run past your general doctor and pharmacist before starting something new.

When tracking and writing up your case study you want to include what oils you selected, why you selected, and what the practical use was decided upon. Then you will want to follow up with your client for aftercare assessments to determine what the client found when using the essential oils, and any emotions, beliefs, judgements or physical irritations that may have occurred. You will use those notes to make sure that you have chosen the right aroma properties and therapies for your clients pathways, and gain feedback for the next time you work together or for the next batch or oils you blend together.

The IJPHA has a traditional layout for creating your case study that I like to follow:

Your case reports will be highly individual, and when shared with your team or others within your practice confidentiality must be assured. Let your clients know of any intention to publish their case, or share their feedback, and let them know that when you share you will not ever share any personal information that would allow someone to recognize who they are.

Client information: State the clients age and give relevant health history; including medications, herbal, dietary supplements and homeopathic medicines. Previous experiences with alternative practices and the purpose for treatment should be clearly written.

Aroma protocol: The aims and objectives need to be stated with clear thought and understanding. The selection of essential oils or hydrolats, which are floral waters, and carrier oil requires both botanical and common name when first mentioned. Make sure you describe why they were chosen and the exact formulation should be provided. Formulations and dosages should ideally be expressed in terms of percentages and if desired also show the drops if determining your cost ratios later. The method of essential oil application must be documented, along with any techniques described, depending on how you are using your essential oils.

The duration of sessions and frequency of treatment sessions should be noted. This will be slightly different when creating your aroma protocol for a client versus a business facility.

<u>Aftercare Client response to use</u>: Observations during the session, if you are working together either in massage, chakras, talk therapy or other treatment therapies. Note immediate client responses and those followed up at subsequent client sessions.

<u>Evaluation</u>: State here the assessment of the treatment from your client's perspective; and what did you learn from your experience. Make sure you that you record the results (or lack thereof) in the session, and the protocol you used.

Be careful about drawing a conclusion or creating a judgement as to what you think you are seeing with your client. Ask them questions, and then ask yourself if what you are seeing is a link between the Aromatherapy treatment and the effect in a single case. Sometimes it is just coincidence. Your record is only a record of your experience so ideally include an assessment of how far it can be regarded as reliable.

<u>References</u>: Where rationale is given regarding essential oil selection, application method/technique selected, the source that influenced your selection should be referenced. All statements, opinions, conclusions, etc. taken from another writer's work should be acknowledged, whether work is directly quoted, paraphrased or summarized.

Your case study should use the Harvard method of referencing. This method is a system in which names and dates are given in the body of the text and the references are listed alphabetically at the end of the report, and you can Google this to get more information.

Notes regarding writing style: Keep your case study sentences short, and use short paragraphs. Make sure that what you have written will not confuse another reader or yourself at a later date. Just like in my salon when I was practicing cosmetology, I had to know what hair color I had used, the formulation, the outcome, and have notes that someone else could understand if they stood into my place to work with my client later.

As a Foundations One Certified Aromatherapist you should create at least five case studies before working with the public. You also would be required to take a Foundations One Certified Aromatherapist test in order to gain your certificate of completion. If interested in learning more about this, please contact me to get started

ABOUT THE AUTHOR

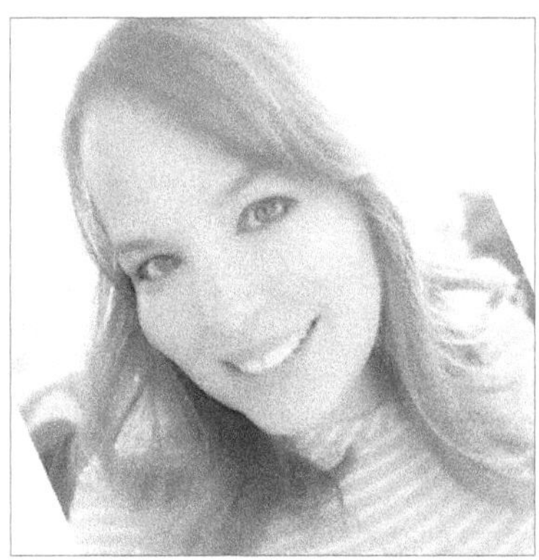

Barbara Christensen is a Certified Aromatherapist who specializes in the energy body connection. She struggled with her health throughout her childhood and early adulthood which lead her to seek out and become a purpose driven alternative expert. Barbara, who also has been trained in the areas of nutrition, energy modalities and anatomy; specializes in whole body wellness, says "My belief is that most of what we are dealing with is passed down and environmental gene expression that can be changed with diet, mindset and alternative therapies." Her expertise has made her a sought after guide for vegan paleo dieters, and those seeking to awaken and create a higher energy vibration.

Barbara homeschools her daughter with special learning and allergy needs, having watched too many kids go through the public system without the personalized support they need. It was the same spark that sparked her creation of the Paleo Vegeo dietary lifestyle and the plant-heavy Ketolicious Reset program. Barbara runs the largest vegan paleo challenge group on Facebook, where you can get support in finding your own path forward. Learn more: www.PaleoVegeo.com

Barbara has found a life balance that allows her to work with clients from all over the world via the internet and online conferencing, for aromatherapy, wellness work and with distance energy models. She specializes in seeking the answers through her claircognizance abilities for mastering wellness readings. Learn more: www.BijaCoaching.com.